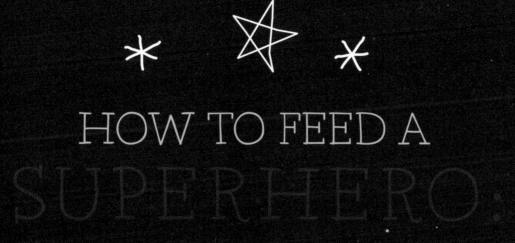

HOW TO FEED A SUPERHERO:

RECIPES FOR THE CANCER-FIGHTING KID IN YOUR LIFE

ADRIANNE SHELTON

Contents

For Taylor.
Our real life superhero.

Introduction

"There is a superhero in all of us, we just need the courage to put on the cape."
– Superman

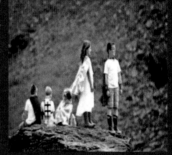

Joel! Get out of there! QuickQuickQuick! The police are coming! 5-year-old Joel was in the campground's outhouse as I saw an Alaska State Trooper car slowly approaching. But since it was first thing in the morning, there was no rushing Joel—not even for the police.

"Is everything okay, ma'am?" The trooper had stopped and rolled down his window, probably because I was frantically talking to an outhouse door. *Yeah, we're okay! My son is in there and he wants to be a police officer and I thought he'd like to see your car drive by, that's all.* "Oh! I can circle around and come back in a minute!"

And he did. Much to Joel's awe and delight, the trooper even got out of his car to shake Joel's hand, give him a "special trooper highlighter," and encourage him in his dreams of being a police officer (or, from that moment on, an Alaska State Trooper).

My most prominent memory of that day was the look in the trooper's eyes when he learned of his fan... I feel like, in that moment, I saw the little boy who dreamed of being the good guy, the hero, the big strong trooper. That's now a look I've seen in Joel's eyes as he uses his special highlighter to write down statements from fellow students on the playground after a punching incident at 0-recess-thirty; or when he passes a trooper on the road and yells "my brother in law!" *That's "brother in arms,"* corrects Nathan... every time.

Six months after our trooper meeting, Joel was diagnosed with cancer.

A friend of ours, a former police officer, reached out to a State Trooper friend of his. "It would mean the world to him if you stopped by in your uniform... maybe even driving your Trooper car. It would make his day." Trooper Hayes thought for a bit. You see, he was a recent cancer survivor. Cancer had been the most terrifying thing he had lived through and he wasn't sure if he was strong enough emotionally to see a little kid fighting that battle.

I'm so thankful he was.

The day we were expecting Trooper Hayes, Joel (only a month into his 3-year battle) watched expectantly out the window for his hero to arrive. There are no words for the excitement that erupted from our home when the expected *one* trooper car turned out to be *eight*.

You see, superheroes never fight the big battles alone.

One by one, the Alaska State Troopers filed into our small living room and surrounded my son with strength and support that he drew from so many times in the years to come. As Trooper Hayes spoke, I don't think he could possibly have grasped the weight of his words. Recounting his own battle against cancer, he connected with our son through a veil of tears.

Trooper Hayes taught us that day that being a hero doesn't mean you are fearless. It means you do what you need to do, even when you are afraid.

To his family, Joel had become a superhero on the day he was diagnosed. But on this day, surrounded by his heroes,

Joel put on his cape.

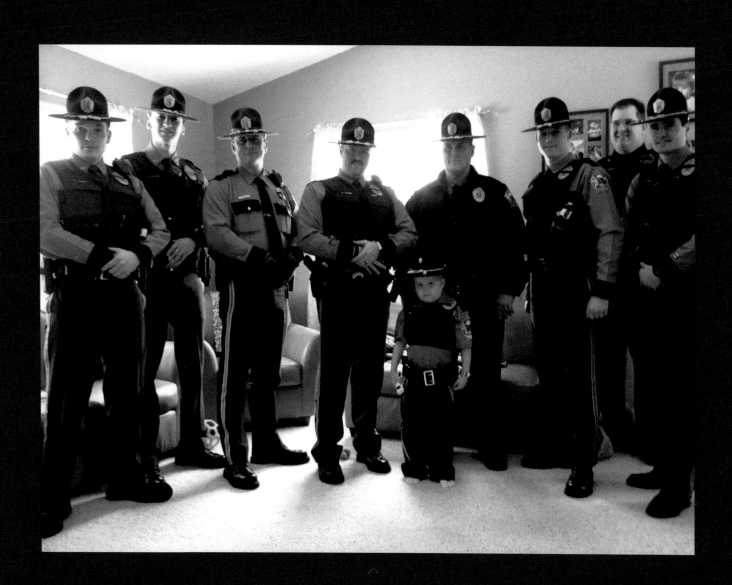

The Purpose of this Cookbook

My philosophy with food is two-fold: **eat a variety of real foods and keep peace above perfection.**

When kids are involved, "eat a variety of real foods" can be challenging. Add the laundry list of chemo side effects to *that,* and the most well-meaning parents can feel helpless. I wanted the food I made for Joel to not feel like an insult added to injury. "Cancer stinks, and now you have to eat this horrible but healthy food while all of your friends down Gogurts and snack cakes." That and, let's face it, no matter how healthy a food is, if your kid refuses to eat it, it's useless! This is where marketing comes into play. Because I know homemade food is constantly competing with colorfully packaged processed food, the recipes in this book are colorful, bite-sized, eye-pleasing, and above all, delicious!

Peace above perfection. That is a mantra I had to adopt during our three years with cancer. **1,000 perfectly nutritious smoothies are not going to cure cancer**... and ordering pizza because you are dog-tired is not going to make cancer worse. So before you go any further into this book, please do me a favor: take that burden of perfection and chuck it into a river. Okay? Thanks!

Looking at the big picture of how your child eats is far more important than a single meal. If your kid drank just one smoothie from this book every day for a week, here is what they would be eating:

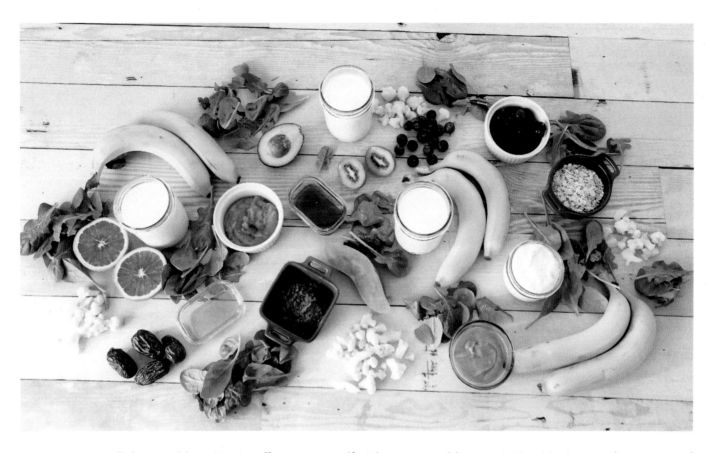

So, you see, small things add up. Don't suffocate yourself with unreasonable expectations, just enjoy the process of taking care of your little superhero as best you can.

Cancer is difficult, there is no way around that. But if passing along my family's experiences and recipes helps even a little, I will have done my job. My hope is that this cookbook benefits the *entire family*. I want kids to feel empowered to feed themselves well as they look through the pages and see themselves as a hero, not just a patient. And I want to give parents and caregivers confidence to navigate the world of nutrition for your growing, cancer-fighting, awe-inspiring superhero.

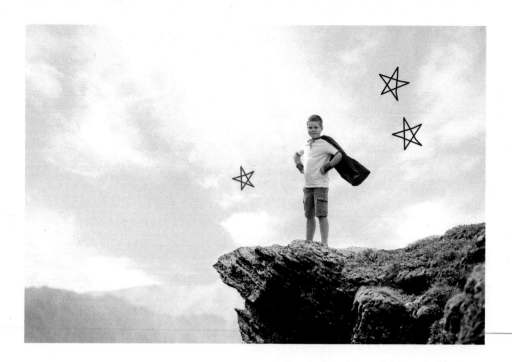

Some Notes About the Recipes

All the recipes in this book comfortably feed a family of five... three of whom are growing boys.

Any recipe that involves baking (i.e. muffins, cookies, bread, etc.) I will double and freeze. The freezer is my friend and it can be yours, too. Any recipe that freezes well will have instructions on how to avoid that horrible, crystalized ice we have all fallen prey to before.

You might notice there is not a chapter in this book about fruits and vegetables... there is a good reason for that! Fruits and vegetables are worked into *almost* every recipe in here, so making a separate chapter felt redundant. That, and there are times during chemo when your kid cannot eat fresh fruit that isn't peeled, or vegetables that aren't cooked, or the acidity burns his or her mouth. So know that I love fruits and veggies. And if it is a time when your child is allowed to have them, there are some fun dipping and dunking sauces listed in here to help make them appetizing to the younger crowd!

The ingredients for the recipes in this book are all things I was able to purchase at my local Costco and grocery store. Nothing exotic, expensive, or complicated here! When I was handed a color-coded chemo calendar and a truckload of medications that come with a biohazard bag, I very much lost the desire to have tedium in any other area of my life—especially in my kitchen! The recipes are simple and the ingredients are easy to find (if you don't already have them).

6

Part I: Setting Up For Success

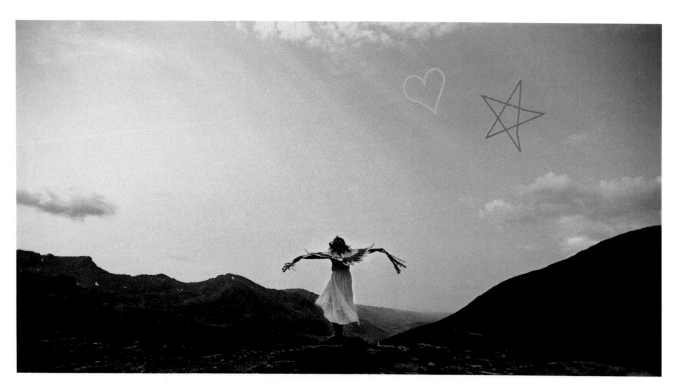

Nutritional Support for Your Cancer Fighter

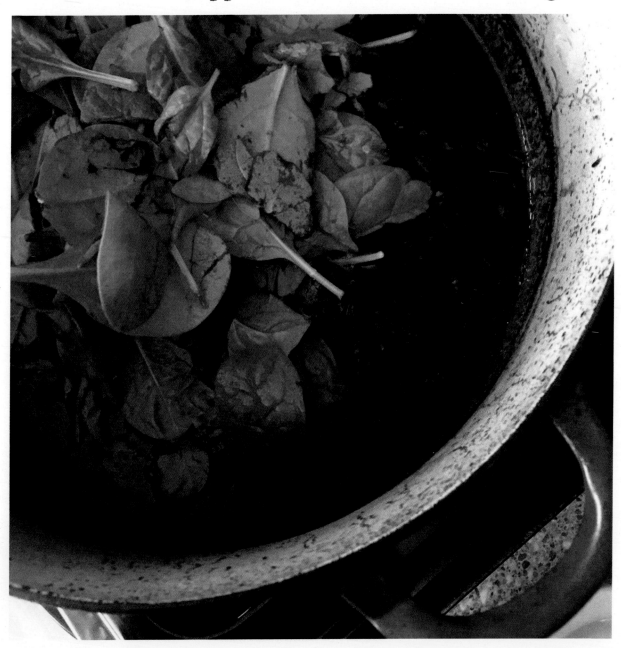

I am a pretty minimal type of gal. I don't like clutter or complication in my space, my processes, and especially in my cooking. Keeping my recipes centered around a handful of simple, but nutritionally potent ingredients keep the reality of homemade food alive in my home.

So, Cancer Parents, you can imagine the reality check I got when Joel's new chemo schedule was handed to me along with a bag of medications, thermometers, gloves…. YIKES. Complication and clutter were my new reality—except in the kitchen. If anything, I appreciated the power and ease of simple recipes built from powerful ingredients more than I ever had before!

Below are the main power players I used as the backbone for Joel's menu and how they supported him through his years of chemotherapy. Keep in mind, the notion of picking apart foods in a scientific manner in order to figure out exactly how they benefit the body is relatively new to the human race. We lived and thrived for a long time by just eating the good stuff… because it tasted good and it's all we had! This is good news, because it shows us we don't have to know the "how's" and "why's" of nutrition in order to benefit from it—we just have to eat it. But if you are a nerd like me who likes to read about food in their off time, this is for you!

Broth

Broth is a good source of easily-digestible protein and minerals. Also, the gelatin that is present in bone broth made at home is soothing to the tummy. Aside from that, 100 years of grandma wisdom is good enough for me!

Eggs

Eggs are a simple-to-prepare, easily-digestible protein. Working hard to chew and digest proteins such as beef or chicken is just not going to fly through certain stages of chemo. Eggs provide a cheap and easy solution for meeting the protein needs of a growing kid whose body should not work any harder than it needs to.

Kefir

I wax poetic about this beautiful probiotic later in the book, so I'll keep it brief here. Kefir is a good source of calcium for growing bones while still being gentle on the tummy, because most of the lactose in the milk has been digested by good bacteria. Those good bacteria then take up residence in the body to keep the plumbing going! Since both diarrhea and constipation pose risk for serious infection in cancer patients, pooping becomes a common conversation topic. Kefir is a great way to keep that conversation on the up and up!

Whole Grains

Whole grains (versus refined, white grains) are full of nutrients including plant-based protein, fiber, B vitamins (thiamin, riboflavin, niacin, and folate), antioxidants, and trace minerals (zinc, iron, copper, and magnesium). Whole grains also contain lactic acid, which promotes good bacteria in the intestine, which in turn supports better nutrition absorption!

Cashew Butter

Just one tablespoon of cashew butter contains 3 grams of protein, and 4% of the recommended daily allowance for iron—that's twice the iron of peanut butter! Butter form versus whole nut is easy on the mouth and digestion. Plus, the natural sweetness and mild scent of cashew butter lends itself well to nauseous patients as it is mostly undetectable in recipes.

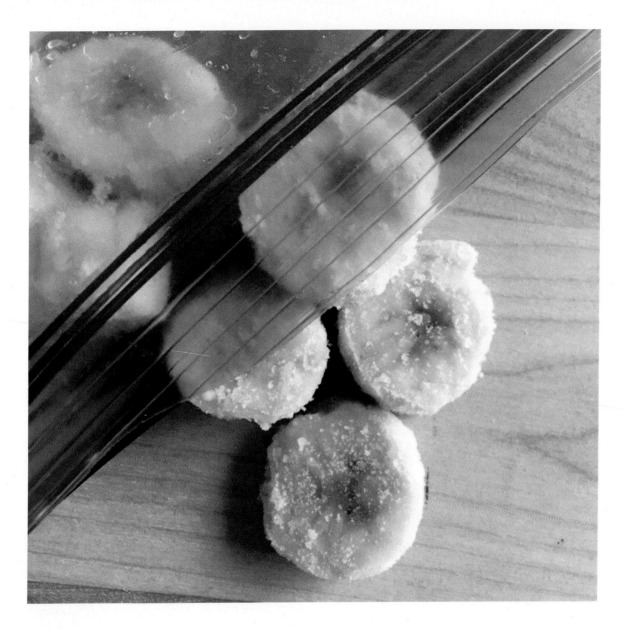

Bananas

Ah, the humble banana! The "middle child" of the fruit world! Aside from being just plain convenient, bananas are an easily-digestible energy source and are mildly alkaline, making them a bit of a natural antacid. Bananas are also a wonderful source of potassium, an electrolyte that helps maintain a proper balance of fluids in the body.

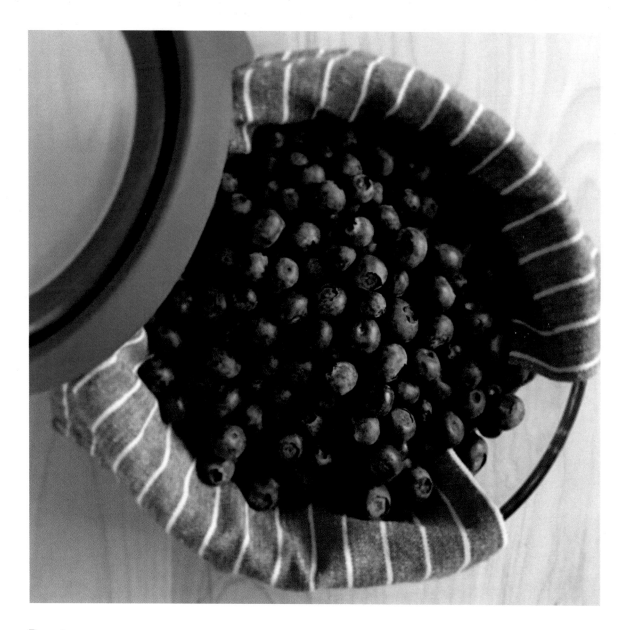

Berries

In the world of unprocessed food, color and flavor are huge indicators of nutrition. In my opinion, there are few things that better pair color and flavor than berries! Antioxidants, fiber, Vitamin C, and folic acid... all wrapped up in a sweet little package.

Butternut Squash

I once heard butternut squash referred to as "the Cadillac of squashes," and for good reason. This bright, silky-smooth vegetable is full of fiber, potassium, vitamin A (for healthy eyesight), and vitamin C (immune system support). Butternut squash also contains a good amount of manganese, which supports bone structure, calcium absorption, and mineral density of the spinal column. If steroids play any part in your child's treatment plan, bone health is a big priority!

Sweet Potatoes

Okay, if you're not already sitting down, it might be time. The list of beneficial nutrients in our little orange friend is a long one.... Here goes! Sweet potatoes are a great source of vitamin beta-carotene (vitamin A), manganese, copper, pantothenic acid, vitamin B6, potassium, fiber, niacin, vitamin BI, vitamin B2, and phosphorus. Phew! Since sweet potatoes are basically the king of vitamin A, it's a good idea to have a little bit of fat served with it, in order to fully absorb the good stuff!

Avocados

Speaking of fats.... Vitamins A, D, E, and K are fat soluble, meaning they actually require fat to be absorbed into the body. Adding avocado to smoothies or meals containing these vitamins will make sure your superhero is absorbing those vitamins to the fullest! Avocado is a monounsaturated fat, making it a good source of energy that will help keep hunger at bay. Along with good fats, avocados contain 20 amazing vitamins and minerals, including vitamin C, vitamin B6 (which helps fight off infection and disease), folic acid, and even more potassium than a banana!

Cauliflower

Cauliflower is a clown car full of vitamins—some of the most potent being vitamin C, vitamin K, and folic acid. What I love about it is that in an easily-digestible form—steamed and pureed—it can be hidden into many "kid-friendly" foods without affecting color or taste. It is truly a ninja vegetable.

Deep, Dark Leafy Greens

Dark leafy greens are loaded with vitamins, antioxidants, and high levels of fiber, iron (for hemoglobin formation and prevention of anemia), magnesium, potassium, and calcium. One of the more significant B vitamins present is folate (or folic acid). Folate promotes heart health and is necessary for DNA duplication and repair. The vitamin K in dark leafy greens protects bones against osteoporosis—which can be a side-effect of long-term steroid use.

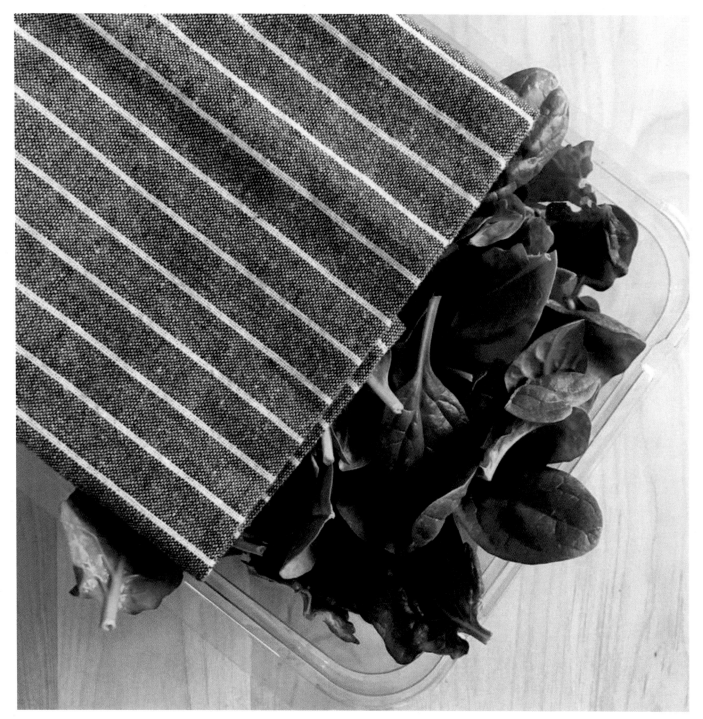

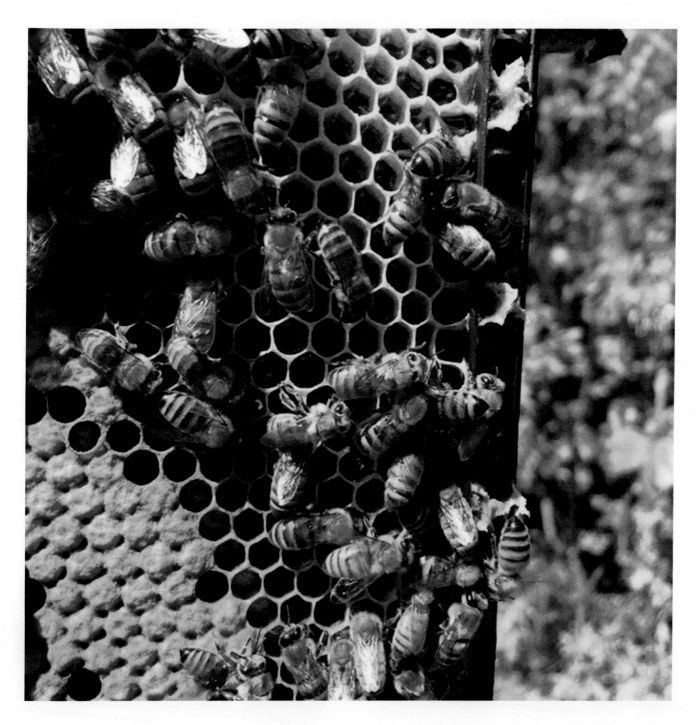

Natural Sweeteners

I have nothing against minimally processed sugar. Adding honey, pure maple syrup, and dates to foods to sweeten them at personal discretion is a far different situation than the loads of added sugar in, oh, *everything* manufactured by the processed food industry! Balance and common sense, that's what I say!

** This was our experience through cancer treatment and was all okay with our oncologist. Always follow your doctor over anything you read in this book. Chemo is touchy and each patient is different. Your doctor knows best! **

ANC: How it Affects the Menu

I remember the first time our oncologist talked about the ANC (absolute neutrophil count). "You're going to watch this number like a hawk!" True story. This particular part of your cancer-fighter's blood work determines your social schedule, neurotic hand sanitizer use, and menu.

The ANC is essentially answering the question "how big is my infection-fighting army?" The normal amount of "soldiers" in this army is 1,500 to 8,000. It is not uncommon for a chemo patient (particularly, patients fighting blood cancers) to stay around 500.

An ANC that is less than 500 means there are not enough soldiers to fight off an infection, should one occur. This means no public, germ-ridden places. No crowds where a person could cough or sneeze. Hospital masks are required when you leave your small, safe place. **And any food that could possibly maybe even slightly potentially bring food poisoning is off the menu.**

When ANC is below 500, avoid the following:

- Fast food or restaurant food that could have been touched or prepared with unwashed hands, or even left at room temperature.
- Any **raw fruits that cannot be washed and peeled**. For example: grapes, berries, cherries, and (at your doctor's discretion) apples, pears, peaches, plums.
- Any **raw vegetables that cannot be washed and peeled**. For example: leafy greens, cauliflower, broccoli, radishes, and celery.
- Deli meats.
- Frozen yogurt or ice cream from soft-serve machines.
- Free samples.
- Unpasteurized juices.
- Raw fish.
- Soft-cooked eggs (over easy, soft-boiled, sunny side up).
- Any food containing raw eggs.
- Soft cheeses.
- Uncooked, bulk-bin whole grains.
- Raw vegetable sprouts.
- Raw honey.

Any recipe in this book that contains ingredients that would be unsafe with a low ANC has had the necessary adjustments noted.

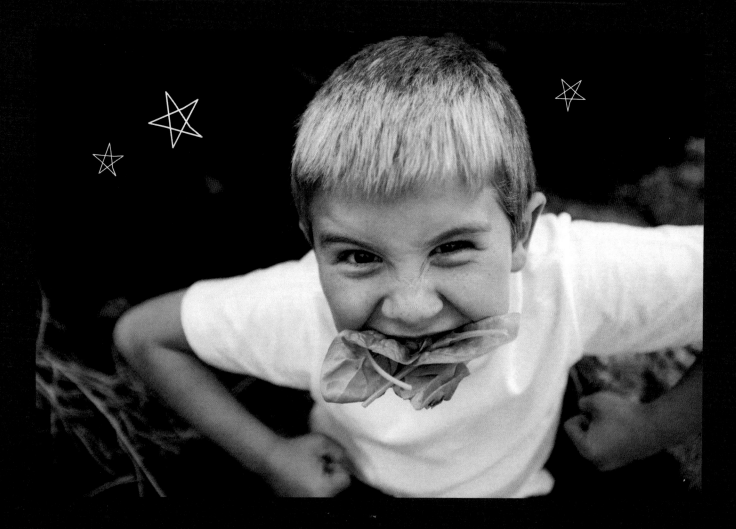

EMPOWERING Your Super Eater

All the healthy food in the world isn't going to make a difference if it sits on a plate, untouched. Having had both the experience of *being* a picky eater and raising kids who are not, I've picked up few tricks to encourage a diverse and adventurous palate.

1. The side-effects of chemo can put a serious damper on even the best eaters. To enhance flavor and encourage appetite, experiment with **The Big Four: Fat, Acid, Salt, and Sweet.** Adding a spoonful of maple syrup, a pat of butter, a sprinkling of salt, or a squeeze of lemon can sometimes overpower the dreaded "pennies" taste that comes with chemo.

2. Nobody falls in love with a food by being forced to eat it, am I right? **Encourage a commitment-free adventure bite!** We always tell our kids that you never know what you will love from one day to the next—taste buds are always changing! We often will give examples of foods the boys currently love (rice, sweet potatoes, salad) that we just hated as kids. "Can you imagine if we had never tried this again? We would sure be missing out on some tasty food…" It is important to emphasize that if they don't enjoy the adventure bite *yet*, they don't need to eat any more of that food at this sitting.

3. **More is caught than taught.** Not being forced to eat a certain food is so powerful when paired with seeing how much mom and dad enjoy it. Many times, my boys will ask to try a food I didn't even offer them (because I was certain they'd never like it). Lo and behold, they will end up loving it. My latest example? Sun-dried tomato cream cheese with flaxseed crackers. My inner-picky-eater-child is *still* surprised by what kids can actually enjoy!

4. Do you believe in love at first sight? I do. Think about it: when you first walk into a cupcake shop, you can't help but get excited about what cupcake you will choose. And this is not because of well-written descriptions greeting you at the door….no, it's the beautiful spread of cupcakes your eyes are drinking in! The same tactic applies to getting your kids excited about eating good food: **hand over the cookbook** and let them have a "first taste" of the pictures. "Ooo, we should make *this!*" will soon become music to your ears! And then….

5. Let your kid be the chef! Aside from the perk of raising someone who will not be dependent on frozen dinners, **a kid can't help but be excited to try something they cooked themselves!** For Joel, cooking became his love during his years of treatment. When he couldn't ride a bike, go to school, leave the house at all, or focus enough to read, he could cook. Cooking became his main confidence-builder and remains a huge source of enjoyment and pride. Fun fact: Joel's quiche is *way* better than my quiche. Just ask my kids. While it is the exact same recipe and I "helped" quite a bit, the boys swear it is better and different when made by a kid! The same principle applies to smoothies around here. I kid you not, one of my boys drank a blended mix of kefir, carrots, and spinach because he was so darn proud of his creation. He said it was the best smoothie ever. I took his word for it…

6. **Talk about it**. *What sounds good? What did you enjoy best about this food? Hmm, I think next time I might change this about the recipe...* This helps kids feel like a part of the process of feeding and eating and can discourage stubbornness around food. A consistent dialogue about food is also really helpful as chemo warps and changes tastes on a daily basis. Talking about what sounds good and what is really icky right now is a good habit for chemo kids. Food is a "safe place" for them to practice talking about how chemo makes them feel. And good communication about their body is going to be so, so important for the rest of their life!

7. **Build a friendly foundation.** Most kids will agree that pancakes are good, so make them green! A chocolate peanut butter smoothie? Yum... Add in some sweet potatoes, greens, and squash! Now, to tell? Or not to tell? That is the question. And the answer is simple: you know your kid best. With my kids, it is always a fun surprise to learn "Whaaaaaat?! No WAY! There was spinach in that?" And, voila! We have a foundation of having eaten spinach without shriveling up in misery.... or whatever it is they are convinced will happen. However, I know kids who would find this to be a deal-breaker. Now that they know there was a veggie hidden in that food, they know to never eat it again. If you are feeding your child through weeks, months, years of chemo, feeding them the good stuff is far more important than showing them they actually ate vegetables. You know your kids best, so take whichever path is right for them.

8. Most importantly, relax! If we were face-to-face, you'd know I was singing "relax." **Good eating habits cannot be forced, but they can definitely be encouraged. And a relaxed atmosphere around food is the best way to accomplish this.** If you are relaxed, a stubborn eater has nothing to be stubborn about. If you are relaxed, a picky eater can rest their fears and find their way. I was a picky eater raised by two picky eaters who would randomly enforce that I eat steamed carrots.... (I still can't handle those). So take my word for it on this one. Once I was grown and married, my husband showed me that it is fun to try new things and that nobody cared if I liked them or not. That is when I finally became an adventurous eater! Take a breath and take a bite, because eating together is a simple pleasure. And as a cancer parent, I know you understand the appreciation for simple, happy moments with your child.

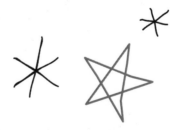

Grocery List and Budget Tips

Here, I have compiled a list of the foods I keep on hand to assure I can make pretty much anything when I have a few spare minutes. Everything in this list is available either at Costco, or at a regular grocery store. Living in Alaska means I don't have a fabulous year-round farmers' market, a Whole Foods, or even a Trader Joe's! What I *do* have is limited time, three little boys, about 8,539 doctor's appointments, and a budget. Buying high-quality ingredients and turning them into simple, wholesome foods is how I keep budgets and bellies happy!

How we keep it affordable

1. **Use it up!** Unless there is some wicked, once-in-a-lifetime, stock-up sale on something like *flour* that will keep a long time and be used for sure... don't buy an ingredient until you are out of it. When the budget is down to $20 left for the week, I'd rather be able to buy milk than say "thank goodness I have 35 boxes of crackers for a rainy day!"

2. **You don't need to buy 100% organic.** Organic food is more expensive than conventional food, no question. If you can afford to buy all organic, that's great! But if you are on a budget like me, do what is reasonable. Michael Pollan says "Cooking [from scratch] is the single most important thing we could do as a family to improve our health and general well-being." Organic ingredients or not, cooking puts you ahead of the game.

3. **Make a list and stick to it.** This is classic advice for a reason: it works. Another benefit to sticking with this rule, cancer parents, is you cut down on wandering time in the store!

4. **DIY.** Even if you are already buying ingredients in place of prepared foods, you can take it a step further. Purchasing less-prepared ingredients is one of my top ways to trim the budget. Making your own kefir is so much cheaper than buying it. Shredding your own cheese saves money (and fridge space!). Skip buying breadcrumbs and use up that heel from the loaf of bread you made earlier in the week! It's a pretty great way to feel like you are sticking it to the man.

5. **Outsource to the internet.** Sometimes, the best deal is online. I use a lot of flour in my life and buying 25 pounds at a time at a discount is often how I purchase it. As an introvert, I always love not having to actually go into a store. As a cancer parent, I loved being able to take care of a few groceries from my phone while I sat in the hospital room for hours and hours. Some great sites for hospital room cell phone grocery shopping:

Vitacost.com

Amazon.com

Azurestandard.com

Thrivemarket.com (Sorry Alaska and Hawaii.... We are not included here—YET!)

Our Grocery List:

Produce (Fresh)

Apples

Bananas

Pears

Oranges

Dates

Avocados

Spinach

Swiss Chard

Carrots

Potatoes

Onions

Sweet Potatoes

Butternut Squash

Produce (Frozen)

Cherries

Blueberries

Corn

Cauliflower

Butternut Squash

Dry Goods

Rolled Oats

White whole wheat flour

Organic, Unbleached White Flour

Cocoa Powder

Chocolate Chips (Enjoy Life brand is my favorite)

Herbs and Spices

Yeast (Red Star is wonderful)

Organic white or whole wheat pasta

Salt (Pink Himalayan Salt is my favorite)

Hemp seeds

Dairy

Whole Milk

Plain, unsweetened, whole milk yogurt

Organic Heavy Cream

Sour Cream (There should be no more than 2 ingredients needed)

Cream Cheese

Butter (Kerrygold pastured butter is the best)

Mozzarella Cheese

Cheddar Cheese (Kerrygold or other "high-end" cheese—shredded yourself--will melt so much better than cheap, pre-shredded cheese)

Parmesan Cheese

Interior Aisles

Organic Tomato Sauce (BPA-free cans)

Organic Peanut Butter (only one or two ingredients necessary)

Cashew Butter

Avocado oil

Honey

Coconut Oil

Organic Beans (BPA-free cans)

Organic Maple Syrup

Organic, shelf-stable mayonnaise (More real ingredient versions are popping

up all the time)

Meat and Eggs

Organic whole chicken

Breakfast sausage (Jimmy Dean Natural has no unnecessary additives)

Organic Ground beef

Organic Eggs

Convenience Snacks

String Cheese

Organic, one-or-two ingredient applesauce packets

Organic Kirkland brand hummus cups

Organic Triscuits

Lara Bars

Resources

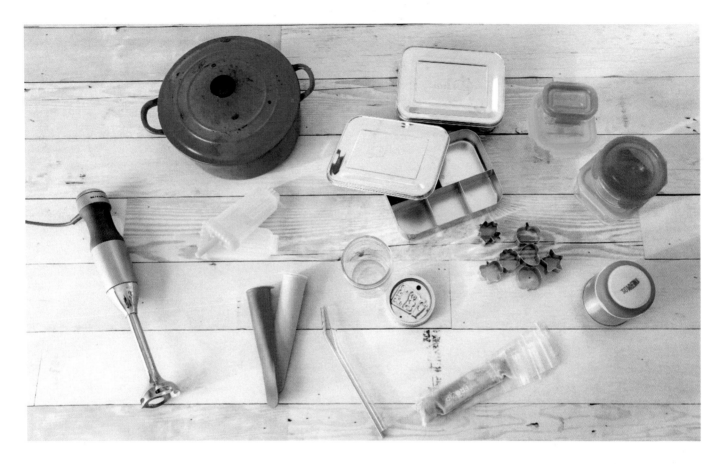

Because presentation is everything...

We all know the saying "never judge a book by its cover." But let's be honest: we all do it-- especially around food. I know that, you know that, and processed food marketers know that. Hence, "kid food" coming in bright, colorful, fun boxes and wrappers. Presentation and packaging are some mighty powerful tools in getting kids to be excited about eating. So instead of feeling defeated by the wolves in sheep's clothing lining the aisles of the supermarkets, let's take a page out of their book!

Homemade food tastes better, no question. But when it comes down to the nitty gritty of actually getting kids to *eat* the good stuff, marketing is everything. Here are some of my favorite tools and supplies to help wholesome food *look* colorful and exciting. These are the exact items I have used for years to make my boys' lunches interesting and fun. One of my favorite memories of this was from when Eric was in Kindergarten. He came home starving because the other kids had eaten all of his food! Lesson learned: sometimes presentation can be *too* powerful!

After Joel was diagnosed, all of these same tricks applied as he passed up pudding cups, tubes of sugar-laden yogurt, and bland hospital food for the good, nourishing foods from home. Shapes, colors, small bites, and fun containers were this mom's best friend. While the tools are a cost up-front, they easily pay for themselves in value over time. I have the same lunchboxes, containers, and tools as I did 6 years ago. Because they last so long, I am able to add fun things to the collection instead of buying new lunchboxes every fall. Not to mention, bringing 5 packed lunches in reusable containers was a HUGE money-saver through our many, many, *many* chemo appointments!

Along with "marketing supplies," I've included a few of my must-have kitchen supplies. I don't like clutter and I don't like washing dishes, so multi-use kitchen supplies are like gold to me. I have even been known to refer to my immersion blender as my favorite child. Too far? Try one, then you tell me.

Silicone smoothie pop molds

Great for yogurts, applesauce, leftover smoothies, creamsicles, and fudgesicles. Available through amazon.com and mightynest.com

Popsicle Molds

Any of the above foods also work well in fun popsicle shapes! Once you start making popsicles, it can be a bit addicting... My boys love the classic shapes of popsicle molds in addition to their usual smoothie pop molds. It's the little things! Available through amazon.com and mightynest.com.

DIY Yogurt Pouches

Use these, of course, for yogurt, but also creamsicles, fudgesicles, applesauce (frozen makes a great popsicle!), juice frozen into popsicles, and leftover smoothies. These are handy when you don't want to have to wash anything out at the end of the day! Available through amazon.com.

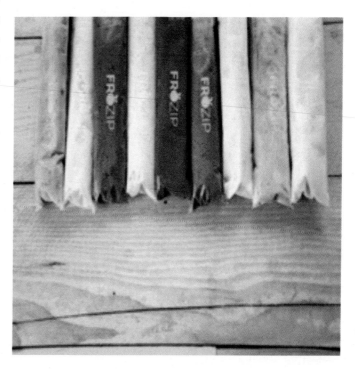

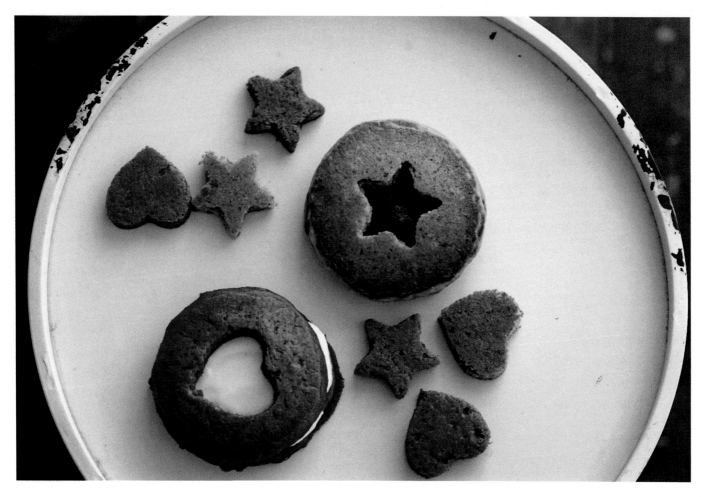

Mini Cookie Cutters

Letters or shapes, these are most often the "trick" to make a food as simple as apples and cheese have a sudden, magical appeal! These are also fun for Sidekick Sandwiches and pancakes). Available through amazon.com.

Immersion Blender

I'm a texture person when it comes to food, so I completely understand when my kids don't like "chunks" in their soup. I'm also *not* a "dishes" person… so I love that this is a small appliance I can toss into my dishwasher. Much easier than a regular blender or food processor! I like how quickly I can smooth out soups, pudding, vegetables, applesauce, and even make mayo at home. This is also a great tool to have around to quickly and easily puree food for sore chemo mouths. Available through amazon.com, Target, Walmart, or most cooking stores.

Stainless Steel Lunchboxes

Bento style lunchboxes are a good way to present a variety of colorful finger-foods! And the stainless steel makes these easy to sanitize and difficult to destroy (*cough* ERIC *cough*). After throwing away two of Eric's destroyed and disgusting lunchboxes in record time, I turned to stainless steel Lunch Bots and never looked back! Available through amazon.com, mightynest.com, and planetbox.com.

Glass Straws

When mouth sores were on our horizon, I ordered these straws. I wanted Joel to be able to sip soups and smoothies, bypassing as much of his mouth as possible. Now we still use them for morning smoothies because, let's face it, drinks are more fun with a straw! Available through amazon.com and mightynest.com and ecojarz.com.

Wean Green Glass Containers

These glass containers come in a variety of shapes and sizes and are a wonderful way to add color to a meal away from home! Easy for kids to open and close and made with shatter-proof tempered glass, I send these with the kids with no worries. Store pudding, leftover chili, soups, sauces, yogurt, baby food… I could go on and on! I started buying these 6 years ago and add to my collection whenever possible! Available through amazon.com and mightynest.com.

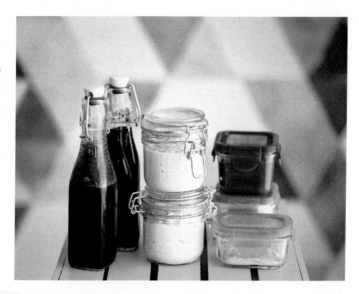

Stainless Steel Drinking Jar Lid

During Joel's hospital stays, I would come home at night and prep food to bring him the next day. Most often, I would make soups and smoothies and freeze them in wide-mouth jars. The next morning, I could pop the frozen jars into a bag and go! Soups would stay cold during the drive and smoothies would be back to the perfect consistency for sipping. This jar lid was the perfect addition to my jar system! Since "hospital Joel" was a slow eater, this kept airborn ickies out of his food while he sipped away over the course of an hour. Available through mightynest.com and ecojarz.com.

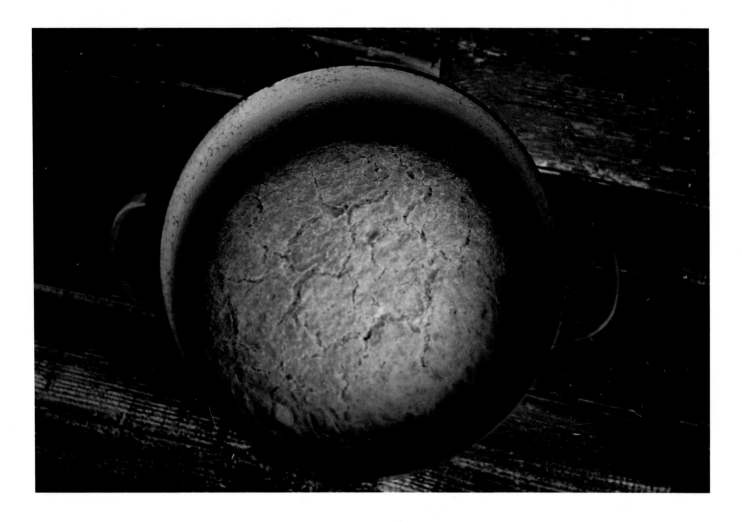

Dutch Oven

For all the things. Soups, bread, frying, boiling, chili, macaroni and cheese... This is the pot/pan I used to replace 4 different sizes of stainless steel cookware. There are a variety of costs and sizes, so choose what works best for your situation. The most common family size is 4.5 – 5 quarts. That is what I have and it is perfect. Available through amazon. com, Target, Walmart, and most anywhere cookware is sold.

Your Half-Hour ACTION PLAN

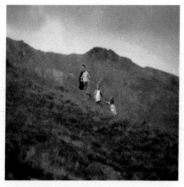

Chemo calendars, doctor visits, hospital stays, and tired kids are all prevalent during cancer, no doubt. What's *not* present? Loads of free time for the caregiver. My number one priority during Joel's years of treatment was being *present* for my family, as much as possible. My number two priority was feeding them well.

Breaking my cooking into half-hour chunks made it possible for me to do both… *most* of the time! There was a fair share of days that drained me to my end, leaving nothing but the sound of a flushing toilet as my mental background noise. Believe me. But as I said before: peace over perfection. Because perfection is not a thing, and crappy days *are*!

On "those" kinds of days, I was glad to have my freezer loaded with wholesome food. And when circumstances allowed for it, I would start and end my day with a half hour in the kitchen. There was something about the quiet of making food that grounded me on either end of a day that felt so full of circumstances out of my control. Therapy and food. You almost can't ask for a better use of thirty minutes.

If you follow the whole plan, in five days you will have chicken, broth, soups, kefir, smoothies, muffins, and frittatas at the ready. Even if you can only fit in one little chunk of time, remember that every little bit helps!

No Time to Spare
(hospital stays, intense chemo weeks)

Day 1:

(30 minutes AM)

Start slow cooker whole chicken

Boil, strain, and refrigerate a box of whole-grain noodles (for use later in the week as macaroni and cheese or chicken noodle soup!)

(30 minutes PM)

Remove meat from chicken

Start slow cooker chicken broth

Day 2:

(30 minutes AM)

Strain and jar chicken broth

(30 minutes PM)

Steam and freeze and/or puree cauliflower

Cut and freeze old bananas for smoothies while cauliflower steams

Day 3:

(30 minutes AM)

Start kefir

Make soup and store in jars

(30 minutes PM)

Put away kefir

Start "There's No-Knead to Fear" bread

Day 4:

(30 minutes AM)

Bake "There's No-Knead to Fear" bread

While the bread bakes, blend and freeze one or two types of smoothie

(30 minutes PM)

Bake and freeze "Lightning-Quick Banana Muffins"

Day 5:

(30 minutes AM)

Make and freeze soup

(30 minutes PM)

Bake "Squashed and Scrambled Egg Bites"

While those bake, blend and freeze one or two types of smoothie

For those days when you can't go anywhere because of a low ANC, have laundry to catch-up on, and want nothing more than to sit and cuddle your superhero while watching Netflix... here are a few minimal hands-on time recipes to make ahead and freeze:

Whole Wheat Bread

Chili

Cashew Chocolate Chip Cookies

PB&J Popsicles

Cheesy Veggie Meatloaf Bites

Granola

Chicken Noodle Soup

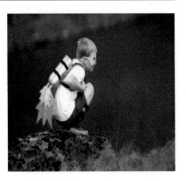

Part II: Recipes

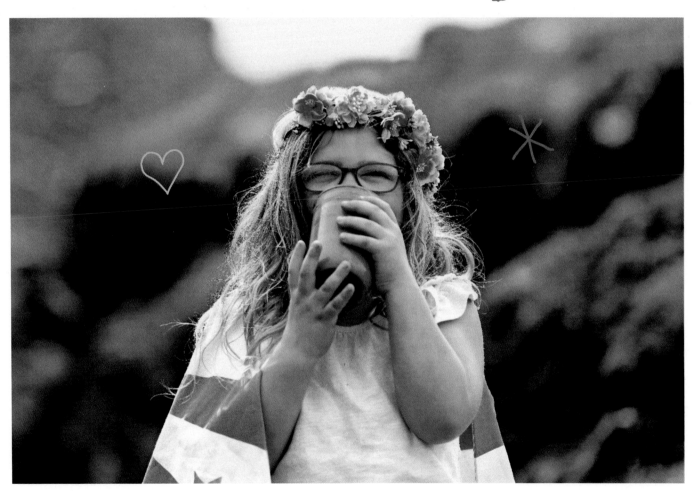

Staples

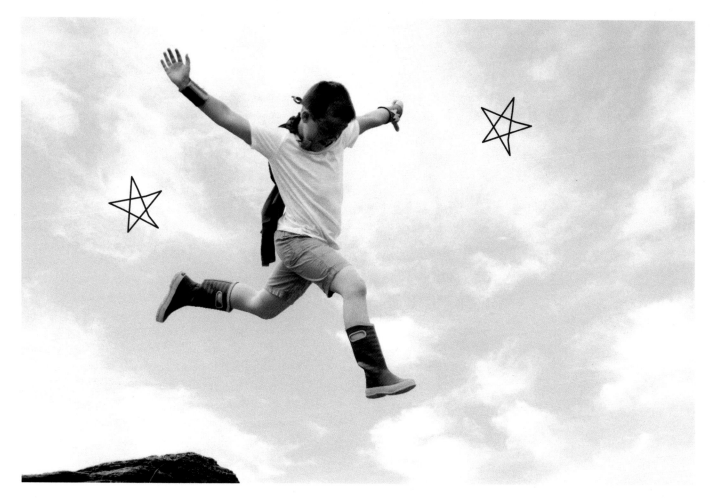

⤜Kefir⤛

Ingredients:

Pasteurized (not ultra-
pasteurized) whole milk

I packet of kefir culture or
¼ Cup leftover kefir

Kefir is our favorite smoothie base! It contains a far larger range of beneficial bacteria than yogurt. And, unlike the bacteria in yogurt that pass through the digestive tract, kefir's bacteria actually colonize the intestinal tract.

You see, the heavy doses of antibiotics used in immune-compromised chemo patients are life-saving—they fight of the infections your superhero's body cannot. But, with the elimination of all the bad bacteria, the good guys get pummeled as well.

Yogurt's job is to feed the already existing gut bacteria, which is great—when they are present! But kefir sends in a fresh round of good bacteria to the ghost town created by antibiotics. This keeps digestion trucking along like it should! One round of mind-blowing constipation after a heavy arsenal of antibiotics showed us the huge importance of refilling the good bacteria in our little fighter. Not only is constipation dangerous to a chemo patient (more infection? No thank you!) but it is a crummy after-party for victory over fever. In short, kefir was a cheap and easy way to keep all the intestinal complications at bay.

The good news: not only is kefir a powerhouse of probiotics, it is the easiest DIY cultured food around. While you can certainly purchase kefir at the grocery store, I find it to be a huge money saver to make it myself—especially given how quickly we use it up!

Some people culture kefir using kefir grains that you retrieve from the milk, store in the fridge, and reuse later. I used a freeze-dried powdered culture, because it saves me some tedium. I keep enough things alive without worrying about kefir grains! I purchased my original culture from cheesemaking.com and have only had to buy it once. The culture is cheap, delivered quickly (to Alaska, people. Alaska.), and the resulting kefir can be re-cultured indefinitely! Amazon is also a great place to buy kefir culture.

Instructions:

1. Fill two quart-sized jars with milk, leaving two inches of head-space.

2. Add half of the culture (or half of the leftover kefir) to each jar.

3. Place the jars into the kitchen sink and fill the sink with warm (not hot-- like you could put a child's hand in it) water, filling to just under the tops of the open jars.

4. Stir occasionally to help the milk reach room temperature evenly.

5. After 5 minutes, remove the jars from the water and cover with lids.

6. Let the jars sit on the counter for anywhere from 4-12 hours. This time simply depends on the strength of your culture. Just tip the jars a little here and there to see how thick the milk has gotten. Once it is like runny yogurt, you're good!

7. Store in the refrigerator for up to three weeks. Remember to save a little bit for the next round of kefir!

 Troubleshooting: Sometimes, the kefir will culture so much that it separates in the jar. While this looks pretty weird, it's completely fine! Just stir it with a whisk (over the sink—it's likely fizzy!) and culture for a little shorter time next round. The more it cultures, the fizzier it will get. But all levels of culture are completely fine to consume.

Makes 2 quarts.

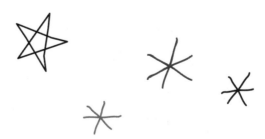

Crockpot Roasted Chicken

Ingredients:

One whole chicken (around 4 lbs)

Generous sprinkling of: Paprika, Garlic Powder, Onion Powder, Thyme, Salt, and Pepper

Simple food at its finest! With a whole chicken's worth of meat in your fridge, the need for drive-thru on the way home from the hospital disappears.

My "Mom Brain" went on the fritz during our cancer years, so I often (read: almost always) forgot that I had made chicken ahead of time. It was such a great surprise when I would open the fridge and see a full bag of chicken-- just waiting for a purpose!

This chicken takes less than 10 minutes to throw in the slow-cooker—it is just so simple. Plop it in the crockpot, season, and be on your way!

Instructions:

1. Remove giblets and neck (if present) from the inside of your chicken.
2. Place the bird breast side up into the slow-cooker.
3. Sprinkle generously with the spices listed above.
4. Cook on High for 2-3 hours or Low for 4-5 hours.**
5. Remove chicken from carcass. Serve chicken immediately or refrigerate in an airtight container for up to a week.
6. Save that carcass for broth!

 **Every slow-cooker is a little different and you know yours best. Mine will cook a whole chicken in 4 hours on *low*— it's crazy hot! You will know the chicken is done when it reaches 165 degrees at the thickest part of the thigh.

Serves 5

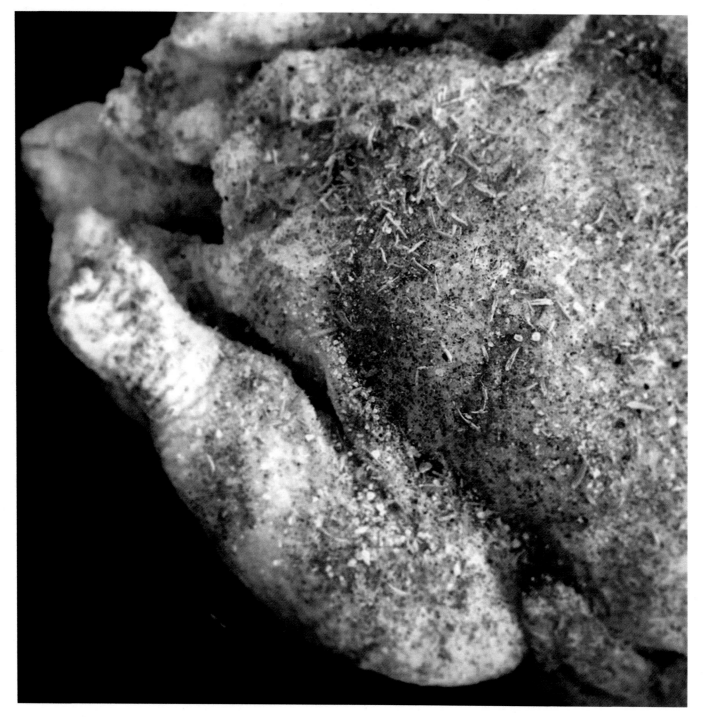

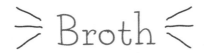

Broth

Ingredients:

One chicken carcass, meat removed

Half an onion

A handful of chopped carrots

I Tablespoon Apple Cider Vinegar

Water

Fun fact: the secret ingredient found in consistently delicious soups is made from garbage. Well, kind of.

I was raised in the low-fat era of the 1980's. This means whole chickens were a rare treat and boneless, skinless chicken breast was all I knew how to work with. Skin? Ew. Bones? Who even knows how to access meat with those things in the way?!

Imagine my surprise and delight to learn I could use those skin and bones to make my own broth. For free. From things I used to throw away. And it's wildly healthy. And I don't have to sit and keep an eye on a stockpot all day long.

This is the original superfood, my friends.

Instructions:

1. After you have removed the meat from the bird from the Slow-Cooker Chicken, place the bones, skin, and odd bits back into the crock-pot.

2. Toss in your onion, carrots, and vinegar. If you have none of this around, don't sweat it! I have made broth from carcass and water only and it was still amazing.

3. Fill the crockpot to just below the top with water.

4. Turn the slow-cooker to LOW and let it cook overnight or at least 8 hours.

5. Strain out the solids and jar the broth in freezer-safe jars (no neck on the jar) leaving an inch of headspace.

6. Use immediately, refrigerate for a week, or freeze for up to a year.

 Quantity varies based on the size of the crockpot.

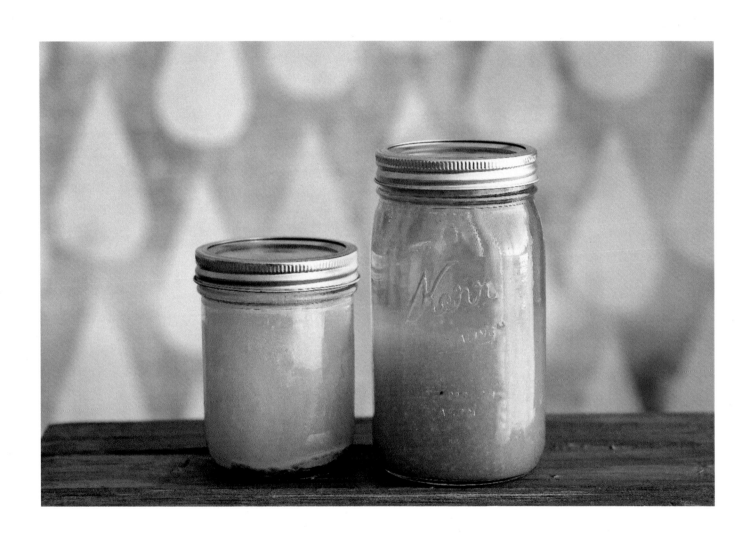

Whole Grain Bread

Ingredients:

1 Tablespoon of instant yeast

2 Cups warm water

1 Tablespoon salt

⅓ Cup avocado oil

⅓ Cup honey

6 Cups flour (any
   combination
   of white: wheat)

Not to brag, but I've made a LOT of pretty terrible loaves of bread over the years... I just couldn't give up my search for the perfect loaf of whole wheat bread! I wanted it to be soft, flavorful, and easy. Too much to ask? Not anymore! This recipe is one I have shared numerous times over the years because I trust it and love it so much. I can't count how many times people have stopped me to tell me how much this bread has changed their (baking) lives! Simple, reliable, wholesome. If you have never ventured into the world of homemade yeast bread, this recipe is the best place to start! I was so glad to have found and tweaked this recipe to perfection before my son got sick... it was a power-player staple for the entire family all throughout his treatment.

A note about the recipe: I have used varying combinations of white to wheat flour here. If you want to have this made, done, and stored in one morning or afternoon, 4 Cups wheat to 2 Cups white is a great ratio. If you are wanting to go 100% whole wheat (which is delicious in this recipe), the bread will benefit greatly from sitting as dough as long as possible. I have started the dough first thing in the morning and fin- ished around suppertime, that works well. But the very best 100% whole wheat loaves have happened after I let the dough rest in a well-oiled bowl covered with plastic wrap in the fridge overnight. In the morning I pulled the dough out and let it come back to room temperature before forming into loaves and moving forward. Time is your friend with whole grains... the more liquid the grain can absorb, the softer it will be when baked!

Instructions:

1. Add all of the ingredients to the bowl of a stand mixer in the order listed above. Alternatively, you can add the ingredients to a regular mixing bowl and knead by hand.

2. Using the dough hook attachment, let the mixer knead the dough for around 5 minutes.

3. Remove dough from mixer and place into a well-oiled glass or ceramic bowl. Cover with plastic wrap and let rise for at least an hour. (See note above)

4. Plop the dough out onto the countertop and cut in half. Knead each half by hand a little to remove any air bubbles.

5. Using a rolling pin, roll one piece of the dough as flat as you can, letting any remaining air bubbles pop out the end of the dough.

6. Tightly roll the dough up like a rug and pinch the seam closed with your fingers.

7. Place the dough into a greased bread tin and oil the top of the loaf.

8. Repeat the loaf-forming with the second half of the dough.

9. Let the loaves rise at room temperature for around 45 minutes, or until doubled in size. The warmer your kitchen is, the faster this will happen.

10. Bake the loaves at 375 degrees for 30 minutes.

11. Let the loaves rest in their pans for 20 minutes before popping them out onto a cooling rack. Let cool completely.

12. Store one loaf at room temperature in an airtight plastic bag for 5-7 days. Wrap the second loaf in plastic wrap, place into a freezer bag (with all of the air removed!) and store in the freezer for up to 2 months.

Makes 2 loaves.

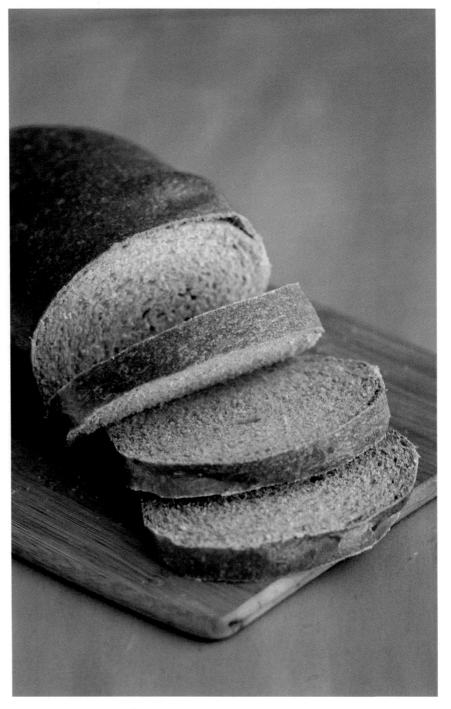

There's No-Knead to Fear! Bread

Ingredients:

1 ½ Cups white flour

1 ½ Cups whole wheat flour

2 teaspoons salt

½ teaspoon yeast

1 ½ Cups room temperature
water

Busy parents, meet your new best friend. This bread was a frequent go-to on nights coming home from the hospital dog-tired. With minimal hands-on time and minimal ingredients, this loaf is still a life-saver when I find myself out of everything at the end of the grocery budget. Pair it with any soup in this book and you've got a simple, filling meal for tired cancer warriors.

Instructions:

1. Mix all ingredients in a medium-sized mixing bowl (not stainless steel) and cover with plastic wrap.

2. Let sit overnight at room temperature.

3. The next morning (or at least 10 hours later), sprinkle a good covering of flour on your counter and plop out the dough. As best you can (because it's pretty loose), shape the dough into a roundish loaf.

4. Plop the dough into a medium-sized, greased bowl.

5. While the dough rests in its bowl, place a Dutch oven with a lid into the oven. Turn the oven on to 450 F.

6. Once the oven is preheated, or at least 20 minutes later, carefully dump your dough into the Dutch oven and cover with a lid.

7. Bake for 30 minutes.

8. Remove from oven and let cool 30 minutes before cutting. If you are headed to the hospital right away, wrap the loaf in a kitchen towel for travel.

Makes 1 loaf

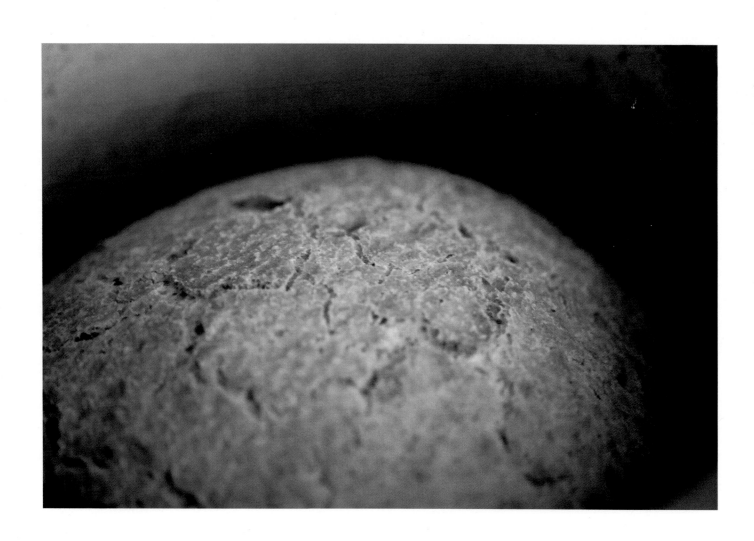

Veggies for Later

When my sons were babies, we were living off of one young teacher's salary. So the notion of buying who-knows-how-many tiny jars of baby food to fill twin boys' bellies was not on our radar! Enter: homemade baby food! Little did I know how handy it would be to have roasting and pureeing mass amounts of vegetables as a skill set 6 years down the road...

In many of the recipes to follow in this book, I hit up basic, kid-friendly recipes with a wallop of pureed veggies. This is not a new idea in the kid food world. I'm sure you've seen some version of this somewhere on Pinterest! Personally, I tried not to "hide" veggies to get them into my boys—I wanted them to know and not be afraid of any fruits or vegetables. But when cancer came along and every. single. bite. mattered.... Well. This was a great way to boost nutrition. While the fiber and bulk of vegetables left whole is good for most of us, the less work a cancer-fighter's digestive system has to put out, the better. Pureeing has done the "chewing" already!

Roasting up a variety of vegetables all on one cookie sheet keeps this a minimal project that will stock you with veggies to boost smoothies and soups for weeks. I freeze the finished veggies in small jars. This allows me to keep a few kinds of jars thawed in the refrigerator to use up over a week's time with nothing wasted from spoilage.

Beets:

1. Scrub 1-2 beets and peel.
2. Cut into halves and wrap both halves together, flat side down in tinfoil, leaving the foil a little loose.
3. Roast at 400 degrees for 45 minutes.
4. Place beets into a small mixing bowl and puree with an immersion blender. Add a teaspoon of water at a time as necessary to achieve a babyfood-like consistency.
5. Transfer to 4 oz. jars leaving ½ inch of headspace and freeze.

For use in: pancakes, smoothies

Sweet Potatoes:

1. Scrub 2 sweet potatoes and dry.
2. Cut each sweet potato length-wise into quarters and paint the flat sides with avocado oil.

3. Place the widest flat side face-down onto a parchment-lined baking sheet.

4. Roast at 400 degrees for 45 minutes.

5. Peel skin off of slightly cooled potatoes and place the potatoes into a small mixing bowl.

6. Puree with an immersion blender, adding a tablespoon of water at time as needed to achieve a babyfood-like consistency.

7. Transfer to 8 oz. jars, leaving ½ inch of headspace and freeze.

For use in: smoothies, pancakes, soups, hot chocolate

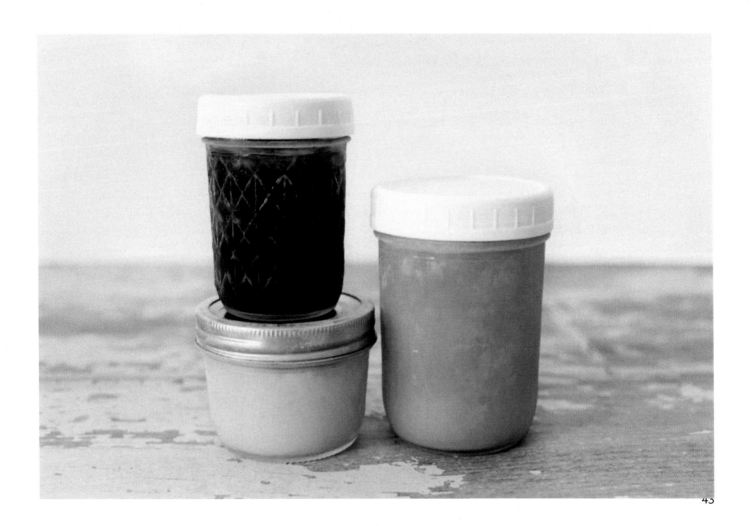

Butternut Squash:

Long, long ago when I was making homemade baby food, I had to make butternut squash puree out of a whole squash. While this was certainly cheaper than buying tiny jars of the stuff, it was tedious to cut and roast a squash and puree it all during naptime! Now, my beloved Costco has organic, peeled, chopped butternut squash fresh frozen into steamable bags. This? This is winning. Now I have jars of pureed butternut squash ready to use and it takes 15 minutes, start to finish.

1. Steam a 16 oz. bag of butternut squash according to the directions.
2. Add the squash to a small mixing bowl with ¼ to 1/3 cup water.
3. Puree until smooth using an immersion blender.
4. Transfer to 8 oz. jars leaving 1-inch headspace and freeze.

For use in: soups, macaroni and cheese, popsicles, pasta sauce

Cauliflower:

Take the easy road here: buy steam-in-the-bag vegetables. Cauliflower is pretty potent while it is cooking and you don't want an already sensitive superhero belly to develop a serious aversion because the smell hung around the house for hours. Microwave steaming cuts down a cook time (and smell time) big time.

1. Steam a 16 oz. bag of cauliflower according to the directions.
2. Add the cauliflower to a small mixing bowl with ¼ to 1/3 cup of water.
3. Puree until smooth using an immersion blender.
4. Transfer to 8 oz. jars, leaving ½ inch of headspace and freeze.

For use in: smoothies, soups, macaroni and cheese, pasta sauce

Once-A-Month It!

Preparing these vegetables to be used in everything possible can be done in one fell swoop. This is how I like to do it for a couple of reasons:

1. I am more likely to add veggie boosts into everyday foods when they are all at-the-ready in my fridge.

2. Mentally, the thought of cooking and pureeing vegetables *feels* like a big task—even though it isn't. At least it feels that way to me... So taking a little over an hour **every few weeks** to fill 8-10 jars with a variety of vegetables really lightens my mental load!

So if an "all at once" method is your bag, here's how I do it:

1. Prepare beets and sweet potatoes for roasting while the oven preheats.

2. Place the foiled beets and oiled sweet potatoes together onto a parchment-lined baking sheet.

3. While the oven vegetables roast, steam your cauliflower, then butternut squash.

4. Puree and jar your steamed veggies.

5. Remove roasted vegetables from the oven.

6. Puree and jar the beets and sweet potatoes.

7. Pat yourself on the back, because you are amazing!

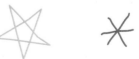

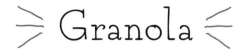

Granola

Ingredients:

4 Cups oats

1 Cup chopped pecans

1 Cup unsweetened shredded coconut

½ Cup maple syrup

4 Tablespoons (half a stick) of butter, melted

½ Cup almond butter

1 Tablespoon vanilla

This granola was a staple in our house long before cancer came along and remains a staple even today. Homemade granola was truly my personal secret weapon to avoid (or at least postpone) the hospital food gut-bomb. With no refrigeration needed, I was able to bring a single serving in a sealed glass bowl in my overnight bag, or just keep a large jar of granola on the shelf in our hospital room. Adding in a carton of milk and a banana from the cafeteria made my granola a filling, stay-with-me meal that didn't leave my belly aching!

Notes: This recipe is forgiving, folks, so don't stress it. If you have enough-ish of any one ingredient, great! If you swap out two cups of oats for sunflower seeds, great! If you want cashew butter instead of almond butter, great! See where I'm going with this? Make it your own! It's pretty difficult to wreck this one. Just don't forget to watch it closely as it bakes...

Instructions:

Preheat oven to 350 degrees.

1. In a large mixing bowl, stir together butter, almond butter, maple syrup, and vanilla.

2. Add in all of the dry ingredients and mix well with a spatula or wooden spoon.

3. Spray a cookie sheet with cooking spray or line with parchment paper.

4. Pour the granola out onto the cookie sheet and spread evenly.

5. Bake until dry and slightly browned, stirring every 5-10 minutes. The time will vary significantly, but takes around 20-30 minutes. Once it starts to brown, it can burn quickly if you aren't keeping a careful eye on it!

6. Remove from the oven and let cool.

7. Store at room temperature in an airtight container for up to three weeks.

Makes about 6 cups.

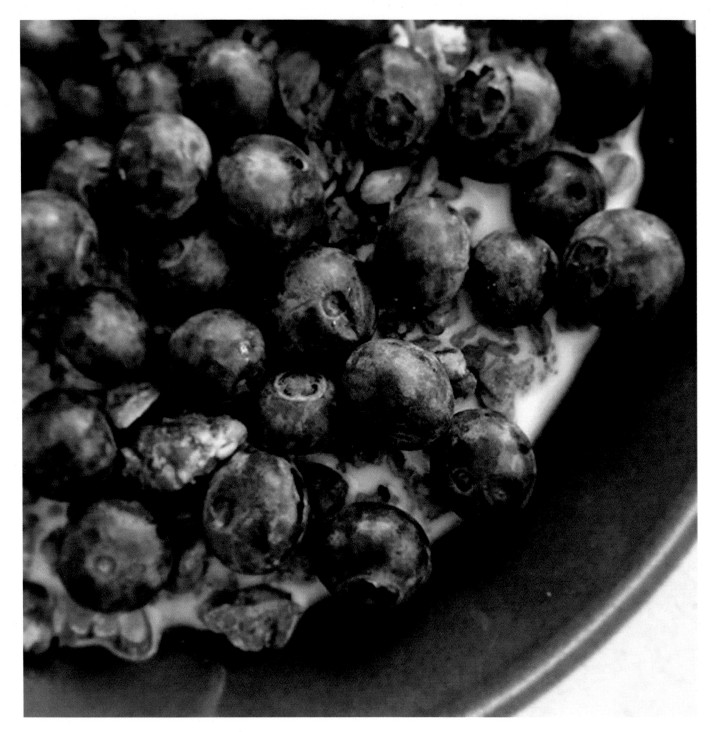

Cold Brew Coffee Concentrate
(The Life-Juice of Caregivers!)

Ingredients:

Ground coffee (I prefer dark espresso roast, but use your favorite beans!)

Water

During Joel's first few months of treatment, I was so tired. [Studio audience: How tired WERE you?] I was SO TIRED, I spent an entire week believing every coffee shop I visited had gotten my order wrong. I'm not even kidding. "Wow, they accidentally used decaf..." Several cups of coffee later, I realized the unlikely odds that every barista in the area couldn't tell decaf from regular coffee. I also realized that I had reached a new low of exhaustion. Yikes. Coffee was about to become an expensive habit....

Cold brew coffee was the answer to all of my easily-solvable problems! With a pitcher of cold brew ready and waiting in my fridge, I could pour two jars of coffee (one for now, one for later) and be off to the hospital in a flash! And, with buying my espresso roast coffee in bulk, the cost was pennies a glass.

Notes: The recipe is for a concentrate, meaning you might want to dilute it with water before adding cream, sugar, or whatever you like in coffee.... I don't dilute. I, however, frighten others with the strength of the coffee I drink. I have one cup of jet-fuel-java first thing in the morning and am good for the day. Do as you like here. Also, because the water is never heated, cold brew coffee is a little smoother and sweeter than hot coffee, so taste before you doctor it up!

Instructions:

1. In a large glass jar or bowl, combine one-part coffee to three-parts cold water. I use two cups coffee to six cups of water, typically, to make enough for a few days.

2. Stir, cover with a lid or plastic wrap, and refrigerate for 12-24 hours. (The longer it brews, the stronger it will taste.)

3. To filter the coffee, place a strainer over an appropriately-sized bowl. Line the strainer with a wet paper towel, cloth napkin, or cheese cloth. Stir the coffee and then pour it through the strainer.

4. Store the coffee in a large jar or sealed bowl in the refrigerator for up to two weeks.

Small Bites to Pack a Big Punch

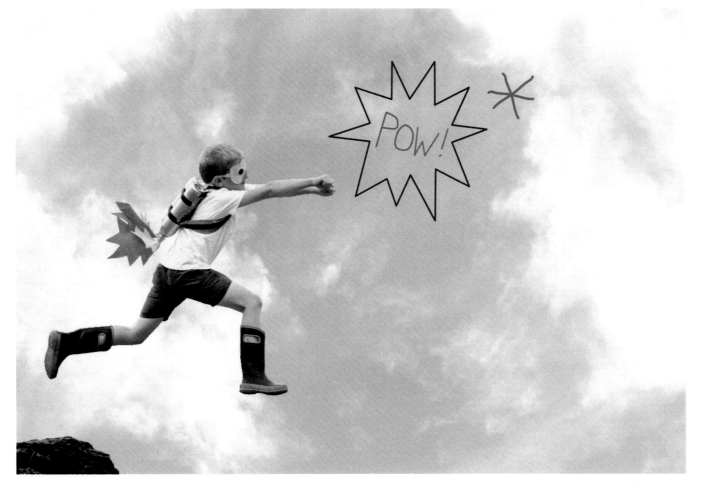

Squashed and Scrambled Egg Bites

Ingredients:

4 Eggs

½ Cup Butternut squash puree

⅛-¼ teaspoon Salt

½ Cup grated parmesan cheese

When every bite counts, these babies pull their weight—and then some. On top of that, they're quick to throw together and bake when you are super-tired at the end of a long day but have nothing to bring to the hospital the next morning.... or so I've heard. Ahem.

Instructions:

1. Preheat oven to 400 degrees F

2. In a medium mixing bowl, whisk eggs and butternut squash until smooth.

3. Stir in the parmesan cheese.

4. Pour into the cups of a well-greased mini muffin tin. I find it easiest to get things even the first time around if I use a quarter-cup measuring cup to fill 3 muffin cups at a time. You want each cup filled to just about half-way. But also, don't spend too much time on perfection… they'll be gulped down all the same!

5. Bake for 10 minutes.

6. Remove the eggs from the oven and let them cool for only 2 minutes or so before removing from the muffin tin and transferring to a cooling rack.

7. Store in an air-tight container in the fridge for 2-3 days, or freeze in freezer bags for up to a month.

Makes 24 mini egg bites

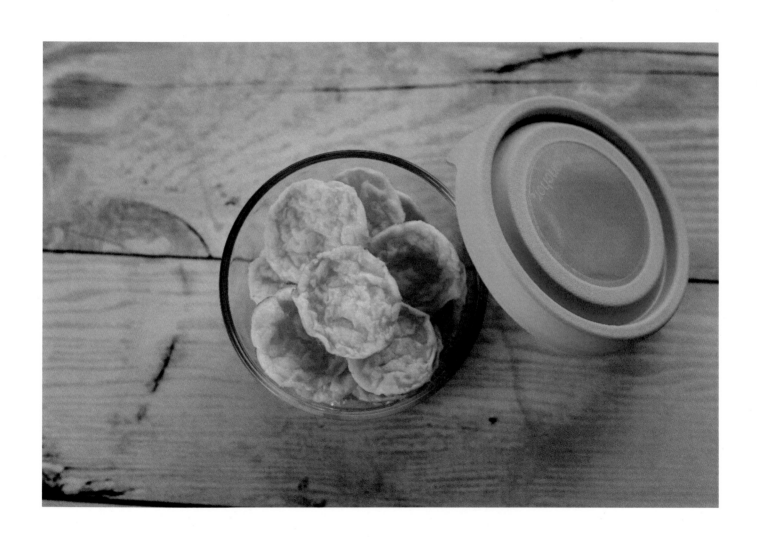

Sidekick Sandwiches

Ingredients:

4-6 slices of whole wheat bread

2-3 fillings of your choice (suggestion box on bottom of page)

Shapes, colors, and finger-sized foods are a great way to encourage even a few bites when the appetite is low. These tiny sandwiches pack nutrition and variety when you make a few flavors at a time. Though, if I'm being honest, my favorite part of these little bites is the smiles they bring when presented as a hospital room picnic!

Instructions:

1. Cut shapes in pairs out of the slices of bread.

2. Using your favorite fillings, assemble the sandwiches.

3. Serve immediately, or store in an airtight container in the refrigerator for up to 2 days.

Makes approximately 12-15 sandwiches

 [suggested fillings box: blueberry sauce and cream cheese; chocolate almond butter; cinnamon PB dip; cream cheese dip and jam]

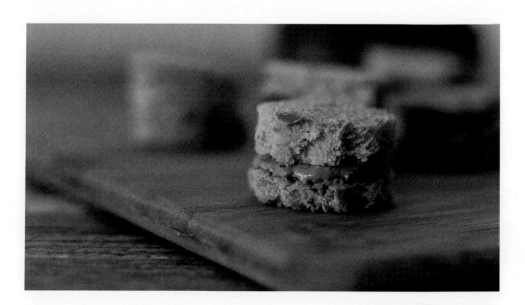

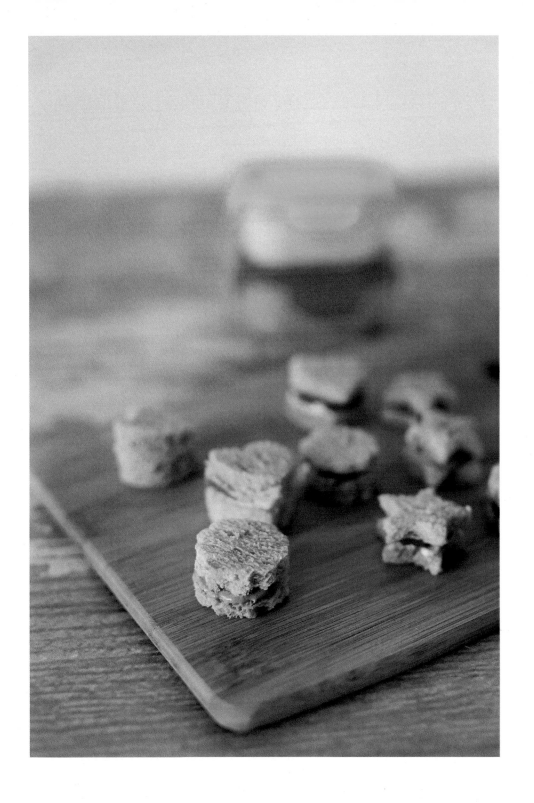

Roasted Sweet Potatoes

Ingredients:

2 Large or 3 medium sweet potatoes

¼ Cup avocado oil

Salt and Pepper to taste

No secret identity is needed for this one. Crispy, creamy, sweet, and savory... nobody can resist Sweet Potato's powers! A superfood that is super tasty—everybody wins.

Instructions:

1. Preheat oven to 400 degrees F

2. Peel the sweet potatoes and chop into ½- to 1-inch cubes.

3. Spread the potatoes onto a greased or parchment-lined cookie sheet.

4. Pour the oil over the potatoes and toss to coat.

5. Salt and pepper and stir again.

6. Spread the potatoes evenly and place into the oven.

7. Every 10 minutes, open the oven, stir the potatoes, and spread evenly.

(This ensures even browning and caramelizing. This is the secret to perfectly browned and crispy potatoes!)

8. Continue roasting and stirring until the sweet potatoes are evenly browned to your liking. The time will vary based on your individual oven, but assume 40 minutes to an hour.

9. Remove and serve immediately or refrigerate in an airtight glass container for up to a week.

Makes 4-6 Cups

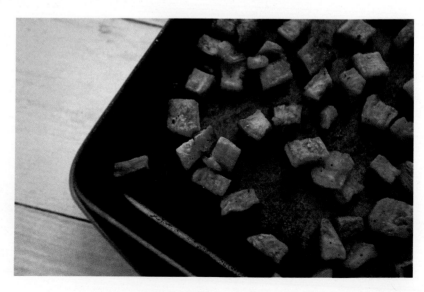

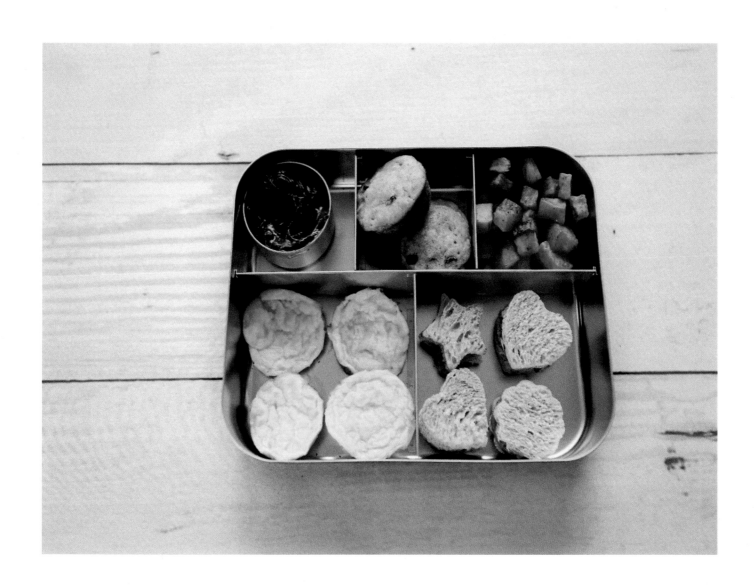

Lightning Fast Banana Muffins

Ingredients:

2-3 Overly ripe bananas

2 eggs

⅓ Cup avocado oil

⅓ Cup honey

1 teaspoon baking soda

½ teaspoon salt

¼ teaspoon baking powder

1½ Cups whole wheat flour

Banana muffins are a familiar and comforting way for your superhero to increase their daily whole-grain intake. Bonus: the simplicity and speed of this recipe make it a great starting point for little superhero chefs! Serve with a good spread of butter or nut butter for a snack that will stick!

Instructions:

1. Preheat oven to 350 degrees.

2. Place peeled bananas into a medium mixing bowl and mash with a fork or a potato masher.

3. Add in the baking soda, salt, baking powder, oil, and honey. Use a whisk to combine.

4. Add salt, baking soda, baking powder and stir.

5. Add in the flour and stir until just combined (a few lumps are okay!)

6. Grease the muffin tin or line with paper cups.

7. Fill each cup to a little over half, evenly dispersing the batter as best you can.

8. Bake for 18-20 minutes.

9. Remove from the oven and let cool 15 minutes before moving to a cooling rack.

10. Store in an airtight bag at room temperature for 3 days, in the refrigerator for 7-10 days, or frozen for up to 4 months.

Makes 12 muffins

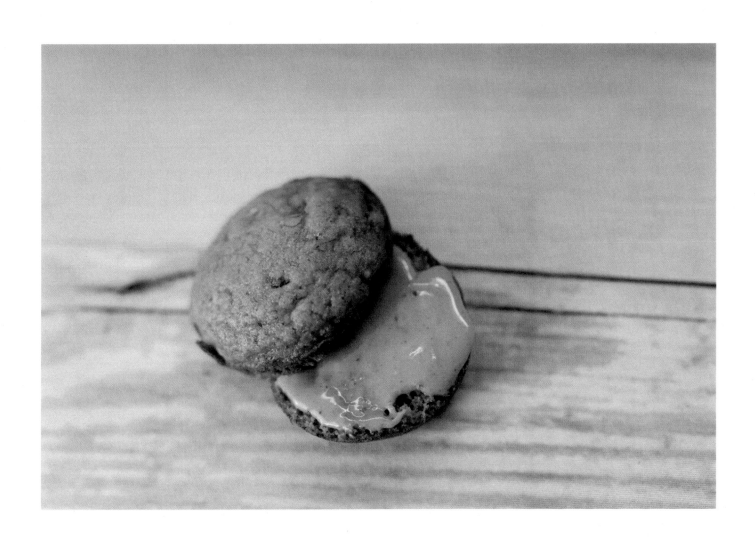

Mini Oatmeal Muffins

Ingredients:

I Cup buttermilk or kefir

I egg

¼ Cup pure maple syrup

½ Cup (one stick) butter, melted

¼ teaspoon salt

I teaspoon baking powder

½ teaspoon baking soda

I Cup + I Tablespoon whole wheat flour

⅓ Cup mini chocolate chips

I developed these little guys during Joel's "frequently in the hospital" days. A bag of oatmeal muffins sitting on the shelf of the hospital room gave all three boys something to grab all on their own when hunger struck. The chocolate chips made the boys happy, the whole grains made me happy. When parenting through cancer, there are no small victories!

We may not be in the hospital much anymore, but these muffins have stayed a regular part of the breakfast rotation—specifically for Monday mornings. Few things get my boys moving and ready for school faster than knowing a plate of these bad boys warm from the oven is waiting for them in the kitchen! Ten minutes of mixing up batter the night before can make me look like a school morning breakfast rock star.

Instructions:

1. In a medium mixing bowl, combine oats and buttermilk/kefir. Stir.

2. Add in butter, syrup, salt, baking soda, and baking powder. Stir.

3. Add in egg and stir.

4. Add in the flour and stir part way. Leave it a pretty lumpy and floury.

5. Add in the chocolate chips and finish stirring the batter, leaving it a little lumpy.

6. At this point, I like to cover and refrigerate the batter to bake the next morning. It allows the oats and wheat to soften and become more easily digestible. However, the muffins *can* be baked at this point if that works better for you.

7. Grease a 24-cup mini muffin tin or a 12-cup regular muffin tin and evenly distribute the batter.

8. Bake at 375 degrees 8-10 minutes for mini muffins and 11-13 minutes for regular muffins.

9. Store in an airtight container at room temperature for 3 days, or freeze in freezer bags with *all of the air sucked out* for up to 6 months.

Makes 24 mini muffins or 12 regular muffins.

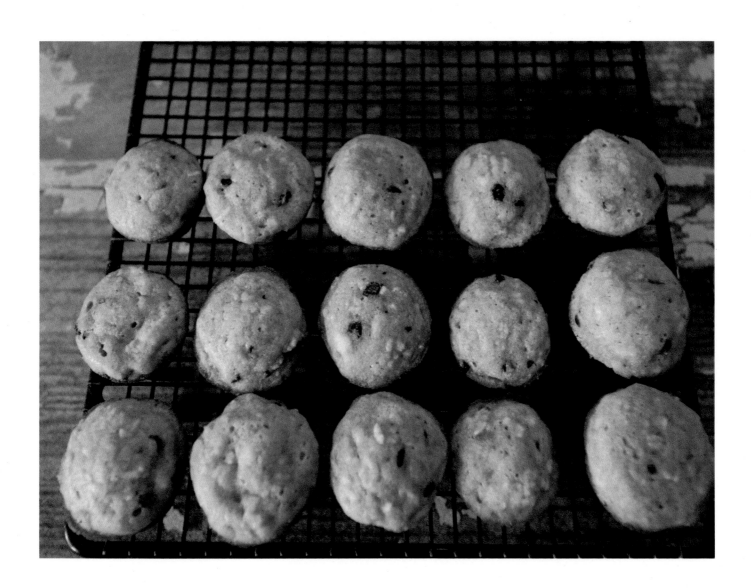

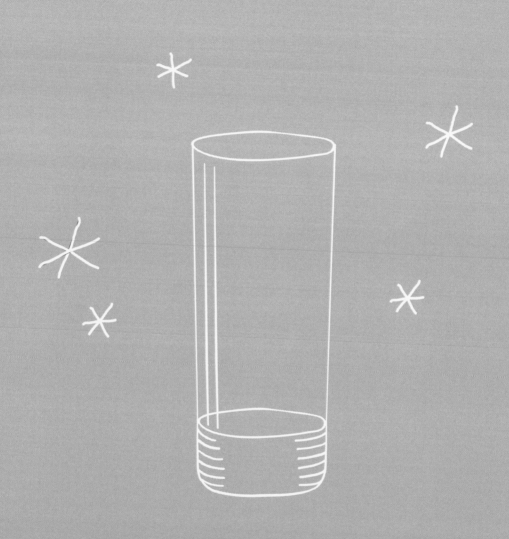

Smoothies

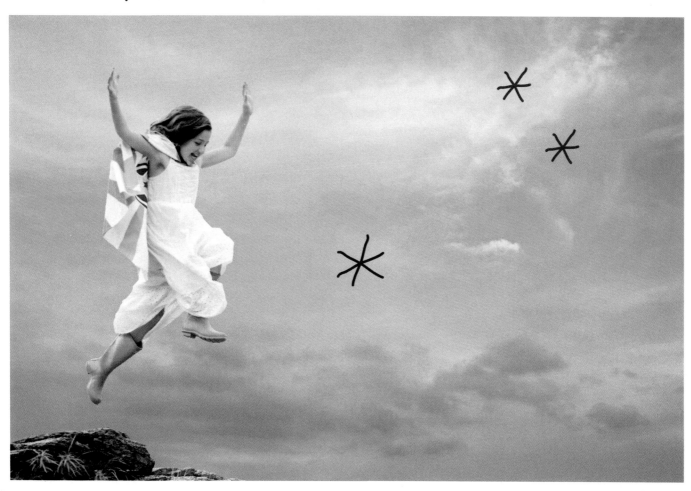

Chocolate Peanut Butter Smoothie

Ingredients:

1 Cup kefir

2 frozen, sliced bananas
(about 1 ½ cups)

¼ Cup pureed sweet potato

1 Tablespoon honey

¼ Cup peanut butter

2 Tablespoons cocoa powder

1 Cup fresh greens, such as
spinach or Swiss chard
(omit if ANC is below 500)

This is the "origin story" smoothie around our house. This was the recipe we pulled out when Eric bit his tongue as a baby and couldn't do solids. It reappeared when Nathan fell on the stairs and knocked his teeth back up into his head. Since we all liked it so much (and I could easily stash greens into it), it became a regular in our breakfast rotation. Later, this smoothie became the answer for how to get calories, fat, protein, calcium, vegetables, and fruits into a brave little boy who had no appetite and a very sore mouth. To keep variety, other smoothies followed. But this one will forever be special as "the one to start it all!"

Instructions:

1. Place all ingredients into a blender.

2. Blend until smooth.

3. Freeze in jars, smoothie pop molds, popsicle molds, or drink immediately.

Makes 2 servings

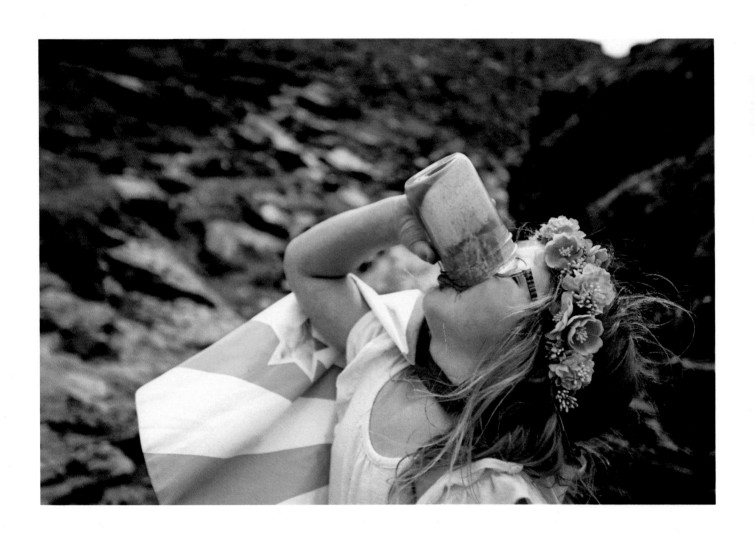

Cinnamon Roll Smoothie

Ingredients:

2 Tablespoons oats

2 Pitted Dates

¾ Cup Kefir

½ teaspoon cinnamon

½ teaspoon vanilla

¼ Cup cauliflower (frozen chunks or puree)

1 Tablespoon cashew butter

1 Tablespoon maple syrup

½ Cup fresh spinach (omit it ANC is less than 500)

During chemo, strong aromas can turn an appetite off, big time. This smoothie pleases sensitive taste buds by skipping the heavy smell of cinnamon rolls and going right to the taste. Oh, and it delivers a handful of vegetables to boot!

Instructions:

1. Pour the kefir, oats, and dates into a blender.

2. Place the blender into the fridge to let the ingredients soak for *at least* four hours, but overnight is best.

3. After the soaking period, add in the cinnamon, vanilla, cauliflower, cashew butter, maple syrup, and spinach.

4. Blend until smooth.

5. Serve immediately or freeze in a jar, popsicle mold, or smoothie pop mold.

Makes 2 servings

Blueberry Smoothie

Ingredients:

1 Cup Whole Milk Yogurt

½ Cup Whole Milk

2 Frozen, Sliced Bananas

⅓ Cup Blueberry Sauce

I knew this smoothie was a keeper when I fed it to my son, Nathan. You see, Nathan doesn't like a) breakfast, b) fruit smoothies, or c) blueberry anything. I always encourage the boys to try new foods, no matter what. When Nathan dutifully sipped his required tablespoon of this new recipe, he fell hard and fast in love. Now? Well, he begs for this smoothie... for breakfast... and he gulps it down every time!

Instructions:

1. Place all ingredients into your blender and blend until smooth.

2. Drink right away or freeze in a wide mouth jar (with 1-inch headspace), or a smoothie pop mold.

Makes 2 large servings

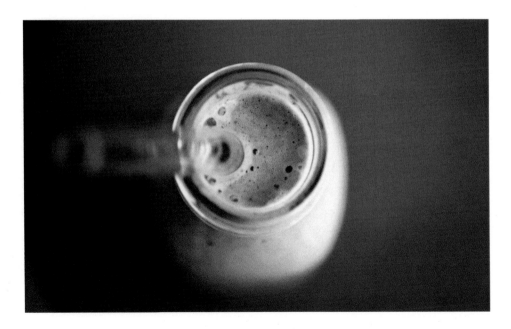

Chocolate Cherry Smoothie

Ingredients:

1 Cup kefir

¾ Cup frozen organic cherries

4-5 frozen banana chunks

¼ Cup pureed sweet potato

½ Cup spinach, packed

1 Tablespoon cashew butter

1 heaping Tablespoon cocoa
   powder

2-3 teaspoons maple syrup

My favorite smoothie in the world. That is all.

Instructions:

1. Blend all ingredients in a blender until smooth.

2. Serve immediately or freeze in jars, smoothie pop molds, or popsicle molds.

Makes 2 servings.

 *Not adaptable for low ANC, so skip this one altogether if numbers are below 500.

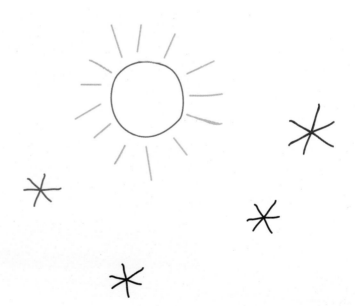

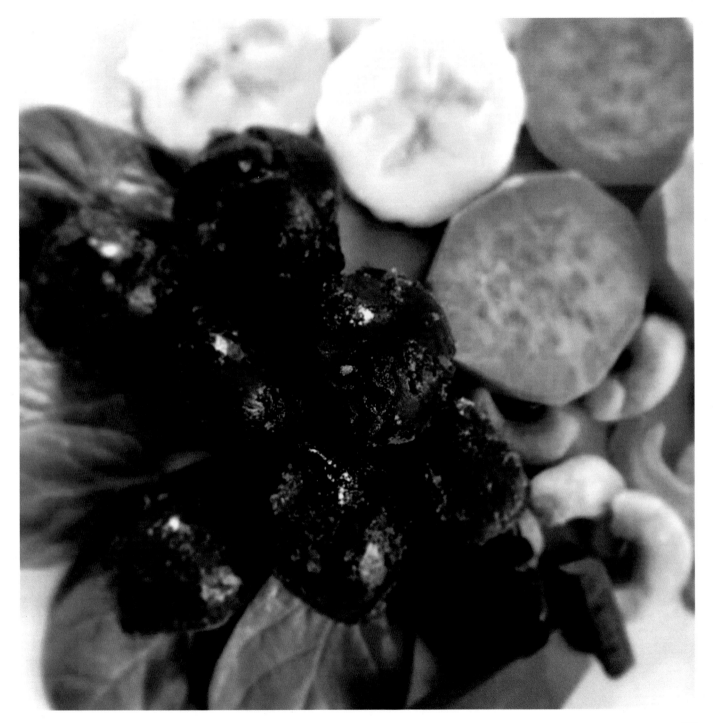

A N (vitamin)C! Smoothie

Ingredients:

One whole orange, skin and pith *cut off* with a sharp knife

5-6 frozen banana chunks

I kiwi, washed and peeled

¼ Cup cauliflower puree

2 Tablespoons cashew butter

¼ Cup kefir

A good squirt of honey

Low ANC means food safety times infinity. Every ingredient in this smoothie is ANC safe, so no adapting (read: thinking) necessary! Bonus: this bad boy is loaded with vitamin C to feed that hard-working immune system with the good stuff.

Instructions:

1. Blend all ingredients until smooth.

2. Serve immediately or freeze in jars, smoothie pop molds, or popsicle molds.

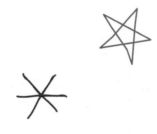
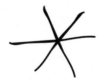

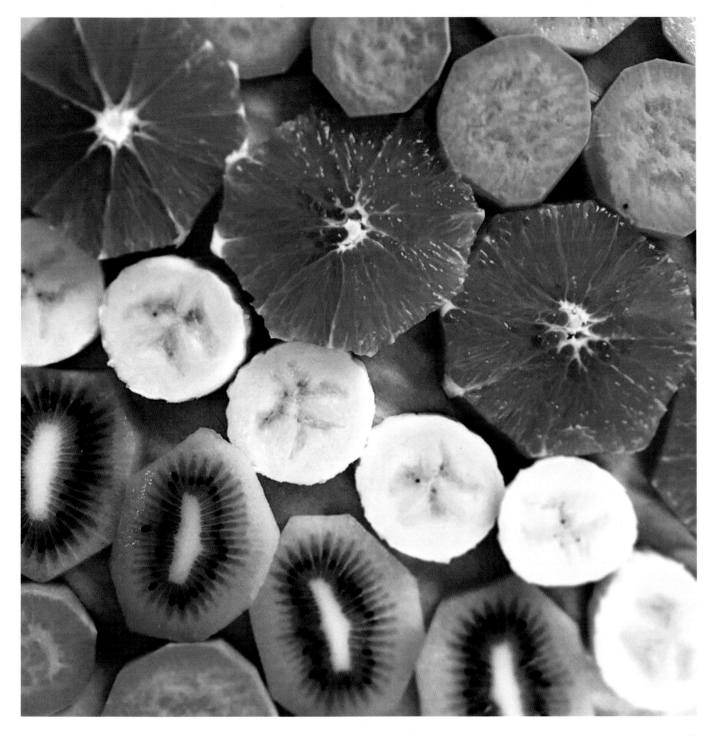

Pumpkin Pie Smoothie

Ingredients:

2 Tablespoons rolled oats

2 Pitted Dates

¾ Cup kefir

I teaspoon maple syrup

3 Tablespoons pumpkin puree

¼ Cup cauliflower (frozen chunks or puree)

½ teaspoon pumpkin pie spice

Thanks to soaked oats and a hefty scoop of pumpkin puree, this smoothie is as filling as its namesake!

Instructions:

1. Pour the oats, dates, and kefir into your blender.

2. Stick the blender in the fridge to let the ingredients soak *at least* four hours, but overnight is best.

3. Add in the maple syrup, pumpkin puree, cauliflower, and pumpkin pie spice.

4. Blend until smooth.

5. Serve right away or freeze in jars, popsicle molds, or smoothie pop molds for up to three months.

Makes 2 servings.

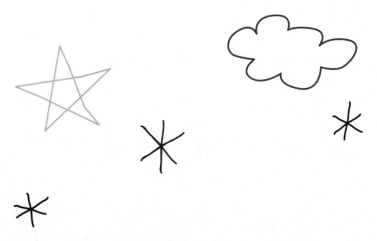

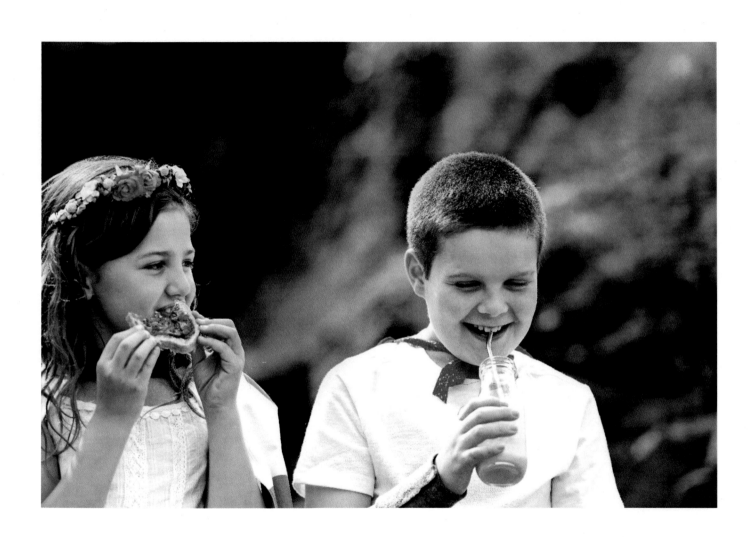

Super-creamy Vanilla Smoothie

Ingredients:

½ of a ripe avocado

⅓ Cup frozen cauliflower
florets (or ¼ Cup
cauliflower puree for
low ANC)

¾ Cup kefir

I teaspoon vanilla extract

I Tablespoon cashew butter

I Tablespoon maple syrup

A great way to get in some healthy fats, this smoothie is gentle to the taste buds and the belly.

Instructions:

1. Blend all ingredients in a blender until smooth.

2. Serve immediately or freeze in jars, smoothie pop molds, or popsicle molds.

Serves 2

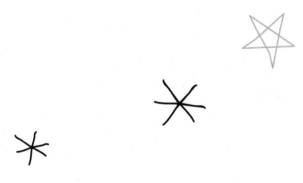

Soups

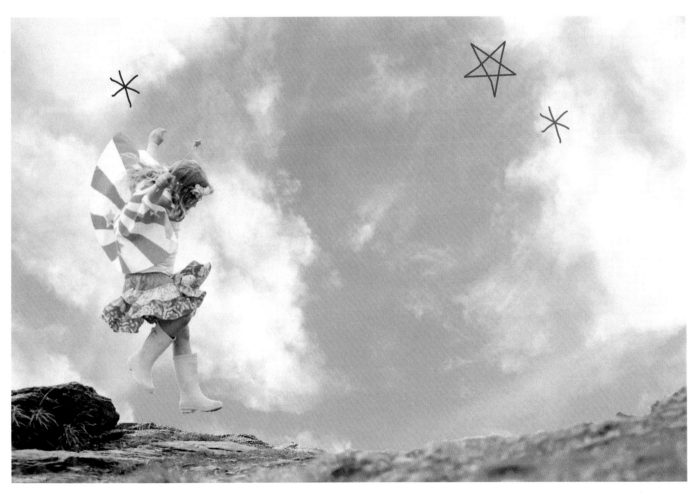

Tomato Soup

Ingredients:

2 Cups chicken broth
  (homemade or store-bought)

1 15 oz. can organic tomato sauce

3 Tablespoons heavy cream

1 teaspoon maple syrup

¼ teaspoon each (or to taste):
  garlic powder, onion powder,
  and basil

Truly, Joel's favorite. Even during the "everything tastes like pennies" part of chemo, this remained his most requested meal (with a grilled cheese, of course!). Forget the canned stuff! This soup takes minutes to throw together and freezes for later like a dream.

Instructions:

1. In a small saucepan over medium heat, combine broth, tomato sauce, and maple syrup.

2. Sprinkle over the top the garlic powder, onion powder, and basil.

3. Let soup warm to a low boil, then reduce heat to low.

4. Add in the cream.

5. Serve immediately or freeze in a wide-mouth jar for up to three months.

Makes 4 Cups of soup

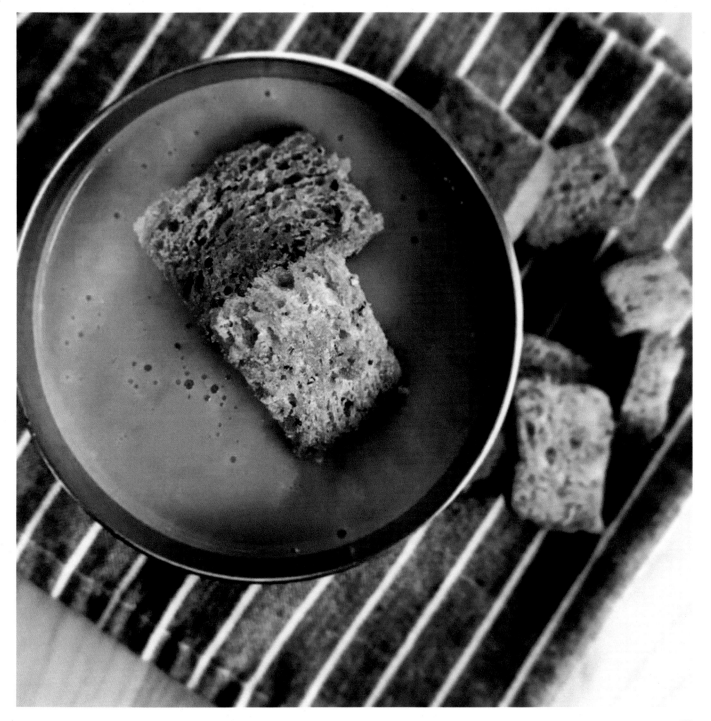

⇒ Potato Soup ⇐

Ingredients:

3 medium potatoes, peeled and chopped into ½-inch chunks

4 Cups chicken broth

I Cup (packed) fresh spinach

I teaspoon salt

½ Cup whole milk

Optional- ⅓ Cup shredded sharp cheddar cheese

This is a great basic recipe that you can soup up based on the appetite and the individual (yeah, I just did that). I left the soup bare-bones when Joel's mouth was sore and his appetite was all but nonexistent. For steroid weeks, I would add in sharp cheddar and some crumbled-up bacon to quell the salt cravings. Now-a-days I meet somewhere in the middle, making a cheesy potato soup that is the perfect something to make a school lunch warm and comforting.

Of all the variations on this simple soup, my favorite involved a gingerbread cookie cutter... Toasting little whole wheat "scientists" to be dunked into the green "gamma radiation" and get turned into "hulking green superheroes," [ahem] encouraged eating and brought smiles. I may have self-fived that day. Just sayin'.

Instructions:

1. Combine potatoes and broth in a medium saucepan and bring to a boil.

2. Reduce heat to medium, cover the pan, and let simmer for 20 minutes.

3. In the last 5 minutes of boiling, add in the spinach.

4. Remove the pan from the heat and add in the salt, milk, and cheese (if using).

5. Using an immersion blender, puree the soup until smooth.

6. Serve immediately, put into a thermos for transport, or freeze in jars (leaving I" headspace).

Makes 5-6 servings

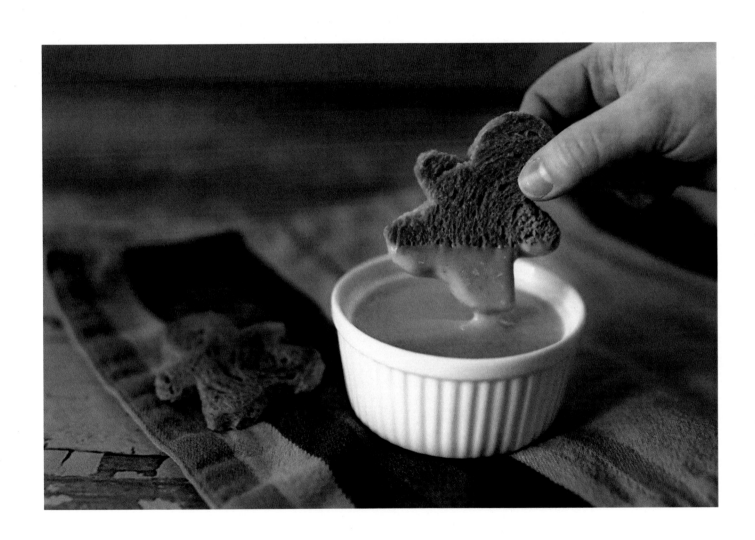

"Choose Your Own Adventure" Soup

Ingredients:

2 Cups chicken broth

1 Cup total of one or all of the following: pureed butternut squash, pureed cauliflower, pureed sweet potato

Optional- ½ Cup packed fresh spinach

½ teaspoon salt

¼ teaspoon onion powder

¼ Cup heavy cream

"Choose Your Own Adventure" sounds way better than "Scrambling at the last minute," don't you agree? We could also call this soup "Luck," because according to the Roman philosopher, Seneca, "Luck is what happens when preparation meets opportunity." See? We're not tired, pulled-in-too-many-directions cancer parents…. We're philosophers!

The preparation here is all of the homemade chicken stock and pureed veggies you already have in your fridge and freezer. The opportunity is the sudden lack of cooking time you may find yourself with that is about to inspire greatness!

15 minutes is all you need to throw together a wholesome soup. Which is perfect timing for hospital mornings and school mornings, alike.

Instructions:

1. In a small saucepan, combine all ingredients.

2. Heat to a low boil.

3. Let simmer 5 minutes.

4. Serve immediately, put into a thermos for transport, or freeze in jars (leaving 1" headspace).

Makes 3-4 servings

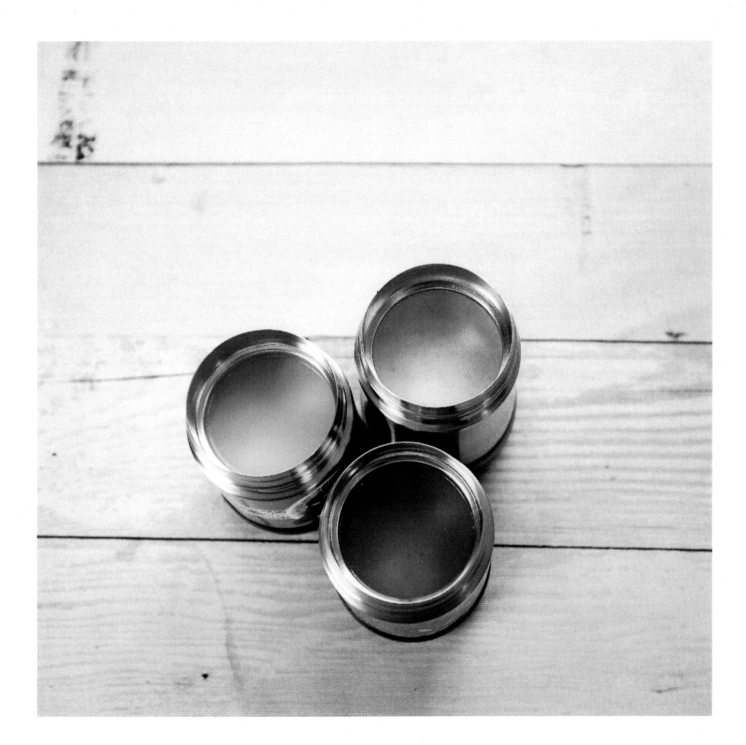

Chicken Noodle Soup

Ingredients:

3 Tablespoons butter or olive oil

3 carrots, peeled and chopped

½ an onion, chopped

4 Cups chicken broth

1 ½ Cups leftover cooked chicken, chopped

1 Cup boiled noodles (fusilli or egg noodles work well)

¼ teaspoon garlic powder

¾ teaspoon salt

It's a classic for a reason! Chicken, vegetables, whole grain noodles, and homemade broth... truly the dream team of ingredients. If your superhero is in a period of mouth sores, this purees beautifully to go down nice and easy.

As I mentioned earlier in the book, having a box of whole grain noodles cooked, drained, and stored in the fridge can make meals like this one even easier. But if you don't have that already, just boil the noodles here while your veggies cook! Speaking of veggies..... why no celery? Well, we just don't like it. But feel free to add it in if you like.

Instructions:

1. In a Dutch oven or similarly-sized pot, melt the butter. Add the carrots and onion and stir over medium heat. Cook, stirring frequently, until the veggies are lightly browned. This takes approximately 10 minutes, but will vary with different ovens, so keep a close eye!

2. Add in the broth, chicken, garlic, and salt. Reduce heat to medium low and cover the pot. Let sit for 5 minutes.

3. Add in the noodles and continue to cook with the lid off for another 5 minutes.

4. Serve immediately, or freeze in jars (allowing 1-inch headspace) for up to 4 months.

Makes 4-5 servings.

Essay: Steroids
A Brief History

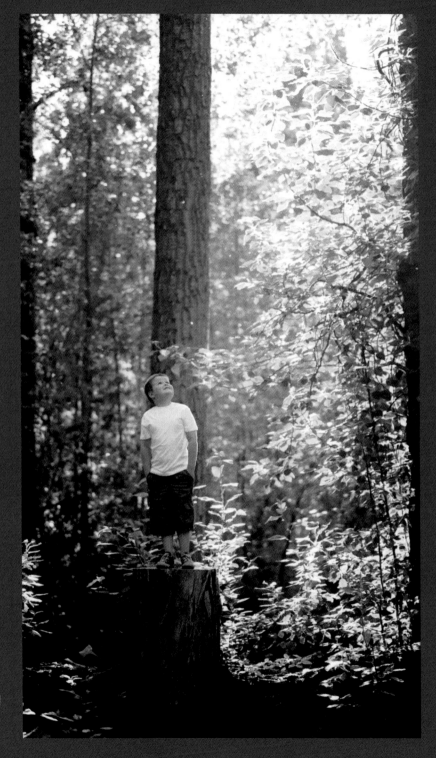

On diagnosis day, we sat down with Joel's team of doctors and got our "game plan" for the next three-and-a-half years. Willy refers to this meeting as "drinking from a firehose." We were given so much information that most of it blasted past us, while the information we *did* take in stung like a beast.

I expected things such as hair loss, throwing up, and loss of appetite. What I did *not* fully grasp that day was what steroids were going to do to my sweet little boy…. If steroids are a part of your treatment plan, you likely know exactly what I'm referring to. We named all of Joel's chemo drugs after members of The Avengers, and steroids were unquestionably "The Hulk."

Mood swings, constant tears, vacant eyes…. and *the appetite.* Yikes.

Once I realized (embarrassingly far into the process) that Joel's "I'm full" switch was absent when steroids were present, I fumbled through more terrible ways of trying to manage his food than I care to admit.

I hated seeing him in constant pain from eating himself sick. And I hated seeing him feel

shame around food because his appetite was completely out of his control.

Joel had been such a good eater before steroids that I didn't want to ruin his relationship with food out of good, but seriously flawed, intentions. Steroids were temporary, but the relationship with food he developed during his formative years would be with him forever.

I decided we needed to treat his Hulk-like appetite like a dog…. Stay with me here! Dogs love to run, no question. So keeping them in a tiny crate (overly restricting food) will make them go bananas. And the first chance they get to run, they'll bolt! However, letting a dog run completely wild and free (no food boundaries whatsoever) can get a dog lost or hit by a car. No Bueno. Enter: the large, fenced yard! **Joel's steroid appetite needed a boundary, but one large enough to let it run.**

Before I go on into the "how" and "what" that we ended up using with Joel, I want to say this: Steroids and kids are rough business. This is what worked for us. Take what works for your family and leave the rest behind! I don't think there *is* an easy, one-size-fits-all answer for how to handle steroids. I only hope that our experience can make things a little easier for someone else in our shoes.

How we Fed "The Hulk"

What worked for us is Ellen Satter's Division of Responsibility. With this feeding method, parents decided the "what, when, and where" of eating and the kids decide "whether" and "how much."

This means, I decided we would have three meals and one snack a day, we would eat at the table only, and I decided what was served. Let's say I serve chicken, bread, salad, and milk. Now Joel gets to decide *whether or not* he wants each of those foods and then *how much* of them he wants to eat. He could, hypothetically, have five servings of chicken, no bread, two bites of salad, and three glasses of milk. Once the meal was done, eating was done until the next scheduled eating time I had pre-set.

This "fence" worked so well for us! Joel didn't feel restricted or shamed for wanting a ton of chicken. And he knew that, while this meal was over, he could look forward to the next one, knowing exactly when it was coming. This might seem strange to anyone who has not seen a kid on high doses of steroids for weeks at a time, but it is mind-blowing watching your previously normal eater become a bottomless, food-obsessed, eating machine. An adult who had to regularly take steroids once told me that it almost physically hurt to *not eat*, even when she was painfully full.

This division of responsibility helped Joel's mind find peace with food, even while his emotions and appetite were raging.

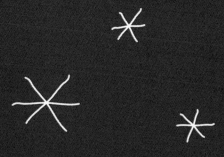

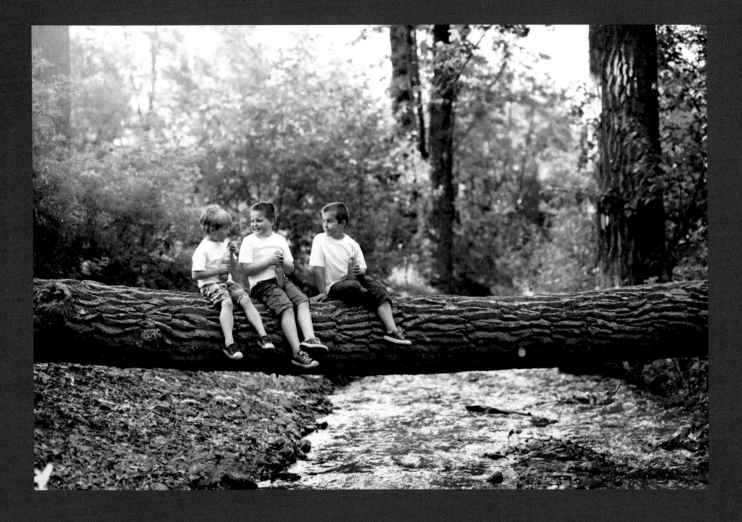

What we Fed

I seriously believe Joel dreamed about cheese puffs and gas station pizza in his steroid-laden sleep! Savory, salty, crunchy foods were the stuff of life to my little Hulk, so I wanted to find a way to honor his cravings while still nourishing his growing body.

[In addition to salty foods, Joel craved a lot of dairy. Later, we learned that steroids can take quite a toll of bone development. It was really fascinating to see how Joel's body craved nutrients he specifically needed at the time!]

More accidentally than intentionally, we landed on a "Mostly/ Sometimes/ Rarely" system of what to offer Joel.

Mostly:

Homemade, flavorful, savory foods. For example: Chili, Macaroni and Cheese, Pizza Grilled Cheese, Popcorn, Cinnamon Roll Milk, and Grilled Cheese with Tomato Soup

Sometimes:

I call these "compromise foods." I am big on making homemade food (have I let on yet?), but there are some things that are just easier to buy, and can be bought relatively high-quality. For example: Applegate Chicken Nuggets, Organic Kettle Chips, and Pirate's Booty (cheese puffs are a steroid kid's holy grail... this provided a happy medium).

Rarely:

Once in a while, we would just go ahead and get Joel the junk food he wanted. As much as we the parents hated when steroid week rolled around, we couldn't imagine how it felt to be the one taking them. Occasional splurges are fun and can give everyone a break. As long as they stay occasional!

And How is Joel Now?

Boy oh boy did we celebrate that last little steroid pill! I loved that steroids helped Joel to be cancer-free, don't get me wrong.... but I hated everything else about them!

Over the first 6 months after he stopped taking steroids, Joel melted away right before our eyes. He had gotten pretty "puffy" (as we called it) and was incredibly self-conscious. He was elated as his pants and shirts were no longer stifling! Now, almost two years later, he looks like himself again, just a little taller (and a whole lot braver).

On the inside, Joel's relationship to food completely normalized. It took a few months, but he settled back into letting hunger and fullness be his guide. Now, he eats a normal-sized breakfast, almost no lunch, and a big dinner. He's found his body's rhythm and it makes me so happy. He also has come to more of an appreciation for how food makes him *feel*. My 11-year-old will sometimes eat too much Halloween candy, but then give away most of his Valentine chocolate because "I just don't feel like ending up with a belly-ache today!" Music to my ears!

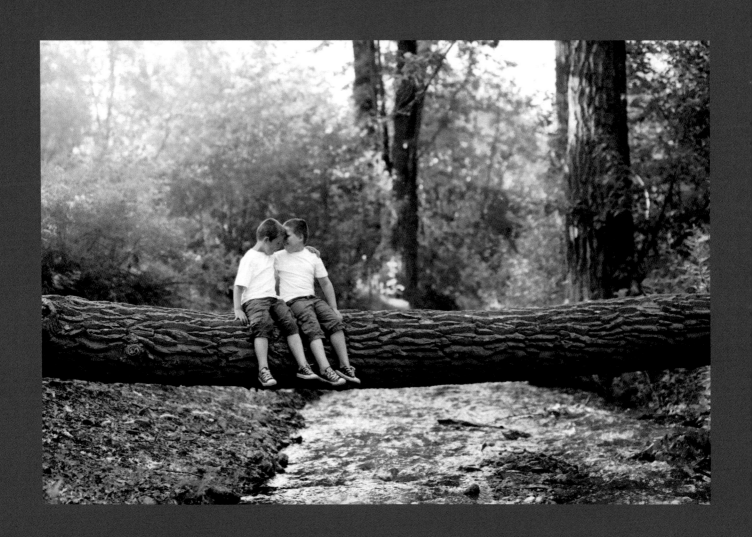

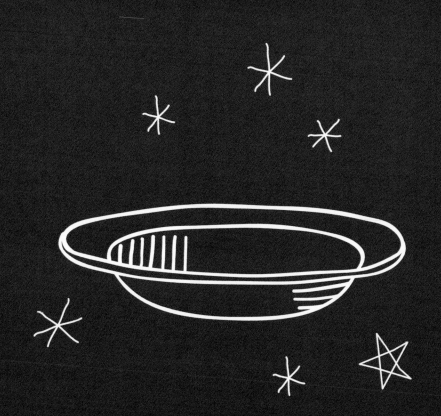

Childhood Favorites

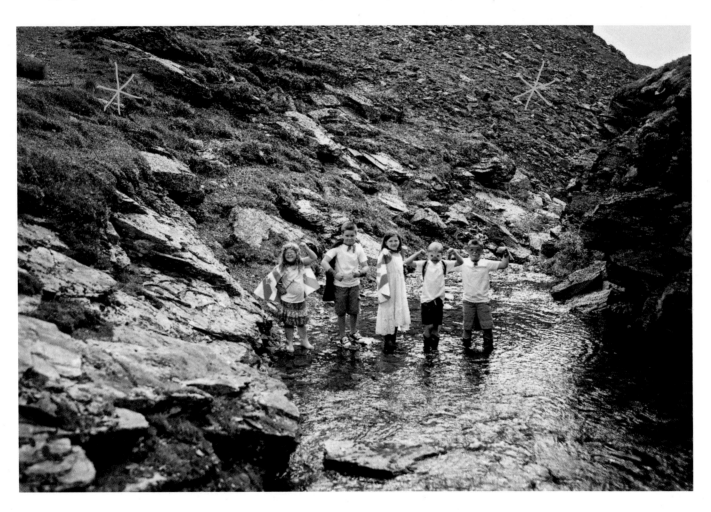

Chili

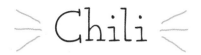

Ingredients:

I lb. Breakfast Sausage (try to find a natural version, i.e. no MSG, nitrates, or corn syrup!)

2 lb. Ground red meat

I teaspoon garlic powder

I teaspoon onion powder

I Tablespoon cumin

I teaspoon coriander

2-3 teaspoons chili powder

I-2 teaspoons salt

3 15 oz. cans organic tomato sauce

I Cup water

3 15 oz. cans low-sodium pinto beans (drained and rinsed)

½ Cup dark or semi-sweet chocolate chips

This chili will forever take me back to "lunch dates" in the hospital with my little man. There is nothing like coming back from a walk with an IV pole down the hallway and warming up a jar of savory, meaty, cheesy chili from home. Not just because it was not hospital food, but this chili let us pretend we were home, snuggling on the couch under one of our cozy blankets.

Now, you may scan the list of ingredients here and say "Uh, Adrianne? Do you just go ahead and add chocolate to everything?" Answer: yes. But this one wasn't my idea.... I read about adding chocolate to chili years ago on a food blog. Trust me on this one. It's the special ingredient you've been looking for. Not to mention, it's a fun secret for the kids to know!

Instructions:

1. Brown the red meat and sausage in a Dutch oven or other large (4-quart or larger) pot.

2. Add all of the seasonings and brown for a few more minutes.

3. Add in the tomato sauce, water, beans, and chocolate chips.

4. Simmer at a low boil until the chili is at a consistency you like. We prefer it pretty thick, so our chili simmers for about an hour, lid partly on, stirring occasionally.

5. Serve immediately with your favorite chili toppings, refrigerate in an air-tight container, or freeze in 2-Cup jars. If freezing, allow I-inch head space to avoid cracking the glass. (We even put some shredded cheese right on top in the jar so it is completely travel-ready!)

Makes about 4 quarts

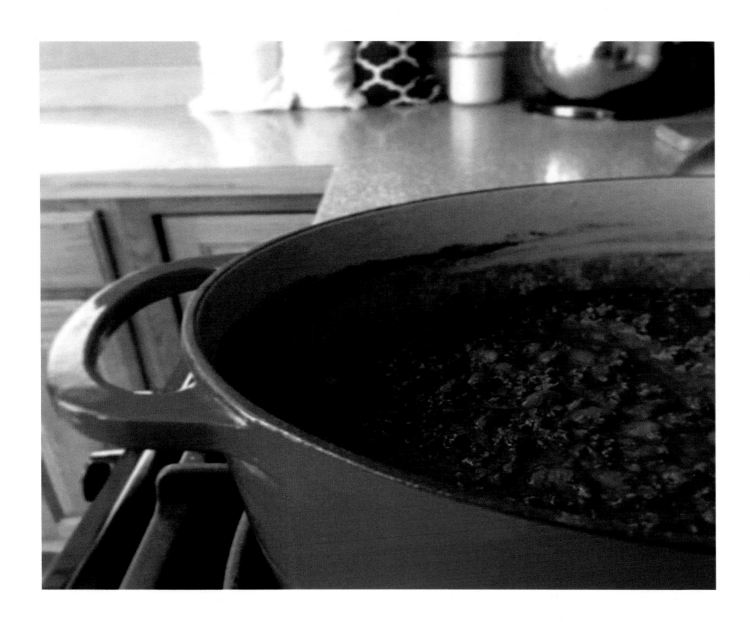

Macaroni and Cheese

Ingredients:

1 ½ Cups whole grain noodles (wheat or spelt)

⅓ Cup cauliflower puree

⅔ Cup cream

1 ¼ Cups freshly shredded cheddar cheese

⅓ Cup pasta water reserved after boiling

½ teaspoon salt

I am a child of the 80's, which means homemade macaroni and cheese never could hold a candle to my beloved blue box. Enter: this recipe. Ten-year-old me wouldn't know the difference. Thirty-[cough]-something-year-old me loves that it is just as quick as the processed stuff, but made with simple, wholesome ingredients (plus some secret veggies!).

Instructions:

1. Boil the pasta according to package instructions.

2. While the pasta is boiling, combine cauliflower and cream in a measuring cup and set aside.

3. Still while pasta is boiling, shred cheese and set aside.

4. When pasta is ready to drain, scoop out 1/3-1/2 Cup of the water and set aside.

5. Drain pasta and pour back into the boiling pot.

6. Add in the cauliflower and cream mixture and stir. Add in cheese and stir.

7. Let the cheese melt into the pasta for a minute and then add little bits of the pasta water (while stirring) to get the desired consistency of sauce.

8. Serve immediately.

Serves 4

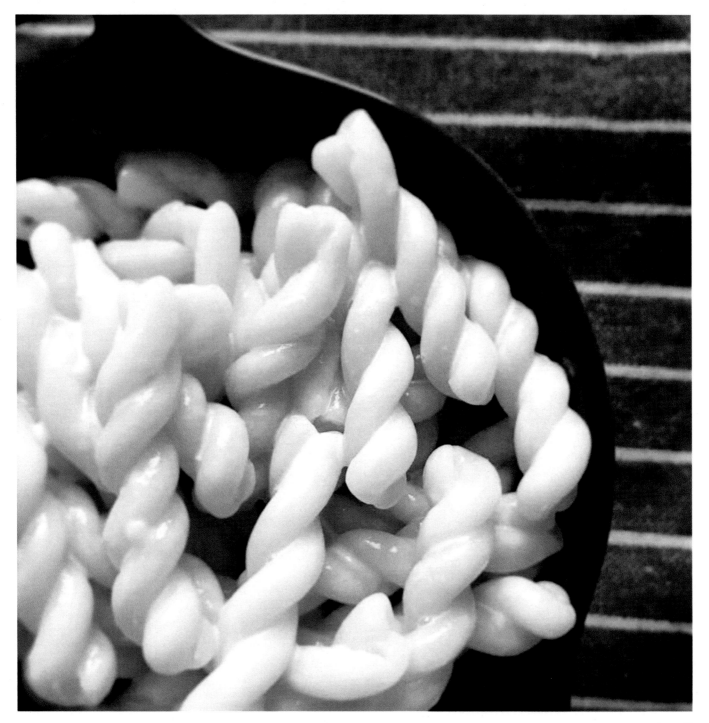

Go-Gurts

Raspberry Yogurt Ingredients:

⅓ Cup raspberry jam or sauce

2 Tablespoons beet puree

2 Cups plain, unsweetened whole milk yogurt

Blueberry Yogurt Ingredients:

½ Cup Blueberry Sauce

2 Cups plain, unsweetened whole milk

Peanut Butter Honey Yogurt Ingredients:

⅓ Cup peanut butter

1 Tablespoon honey

¼ Cup butternut squash puree

2 Cups plain, unsweetened whole milk yogurt

Banana Cinnamon Yogurt Ingredients:

1 very ripe banana, mashed or pureed

¼ teaspoon cinnamon

¼ Cup sweet potato puree

2 Cups plain, unsweetened whole milk yogurt

It may sound strange, but Joel had some serious yogurt envy during his first few hospital visits... There's just something about colorful yogurt that is packaged in tube form that totally trumps a jar of yogurt from home. "I wish I could have a go-gurt like all the other patients do.... [puppy dog eyes]" Challenge accepted! Well, not so much a challenge as a quick "trip" to Amazon on my phone while Joel napped in his hospital bed. A few days and a few dollars later, I had a package of 125 empty "make your own yogurt in a tube" bags in my mailbox. Easy peasy. Not only was this so much cheaper than buying organic yogurt tubes from the store (or even regular, for that matter), but I was able to use only wholesome ingredients that would feed my little superhero's body well.

Using already prepared veggies and sauces, or even just a jar of your favorite organic jam, these come together really quickly and have about 1 million fewer additives and grams of sugar than the pre-packaged stuff.

Instructions:

1. Combine all ingredients in a small bowl, preferably one that pours well.
2. Stir!
3. Pour into yogurt tube bags and seal.
4. Store in the fridge for 2 weeks, or freeze and pull out as needed.

 ** If you have a kid who doesn't care at all about yogurt in a tube versus yogurt in a bowl, simply store the yogurt in small jars. Smoothie pop molds also work well here as a reusable option.

Servings Vary

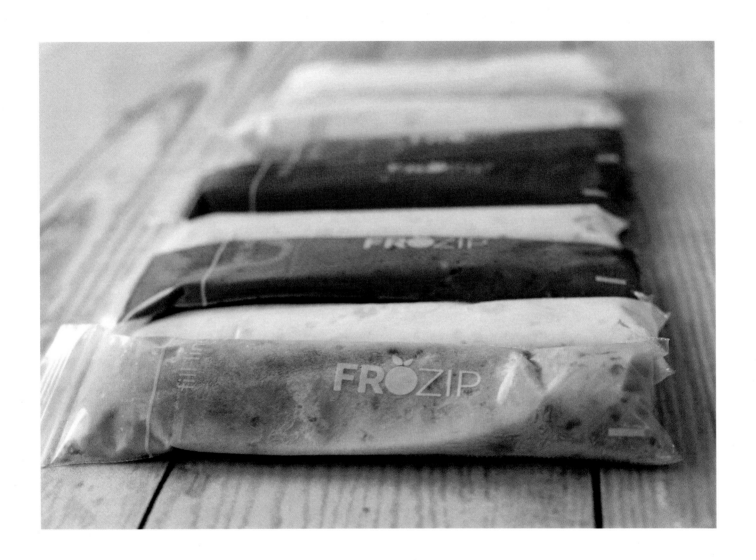

Pancakes with a PUNCH!

Ingredients:

1 Cup kefir or whole milk

1 egg

⅓ cup old fashioned oats

¾ Cup whole wheat flour

1 Tablespoon avocado oil

1 Tablespoon honey

2 teaspoons baking powder

½ teaspoon salt

One of the following- ⅓ Cup beet puree, ⅓ Cup sweet potato puree, or 1 packed cup of fresh spinach

Pancakes were one of the first foods I "greened," and are still one of my favorites to play with. Putting butter and syrup on a food can make just about any kid forget to freak out about the fact that it's green. Or pink. Or orange.

Vegetables and whole grains in a kid-friendly package... yes, please!

I will make a batch of each three colors to freeze, so I can pull out and serve a rainbow of pancakes for a breakfast stack, or as a fun sandwich for lunch.

Instructions:

1. In a blender, combine all of the ingredients except the flour.

2. Blend until smooth, about 2 minutes.

3. Add the flour and pulse until just combined.

4. Let the batter rest for about 5-10 minutes while you pre-heat a skillet to medium heat. This resting period allows the wheat and oats to absorb some of the liquid from the batter, making for softer pancakes.

5. Pour the pancake batter onto a skillet at whatever size you want! Silver dollar all the way to plate-sized work fine.

6. Once the pancakes look bubbly with dry edges, flip and cook for 1-2 more minutes.

7. Serve pancakes immediately, or prepare for freezing.

8. To freeze pancakes, first let them cool on a rack.

9. Once cool, place pancakes in a freezer bag, slightly overlapping each other. This allows for fitting a good amount into the bag, while making it easy to pull them out for use one-at-a-time!

10. Remove all air from the bag, add another bag and remove all the air.

11. Freeze! These keep well frozen for up to 3 months.

Makes 7-10 pancakes

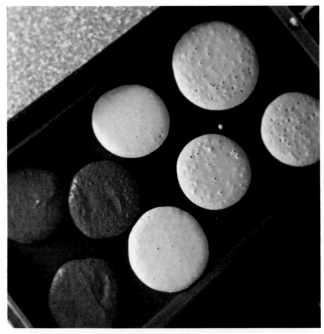
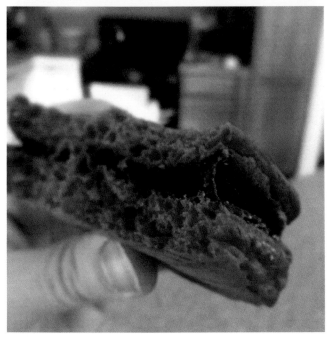
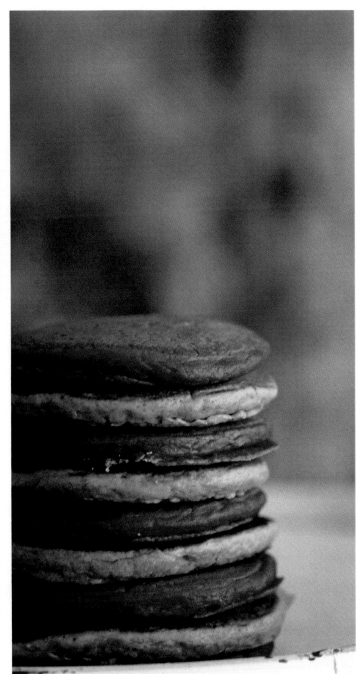

⇒ Quick and Easy Popcorn ⇐

Ingredients:

1 Tablespoon coconut oil

⅓ Cup popcorn kernels

Salt to taste

This popcorn was my inexpensive way to feed the salt-and-crunch-craving beast that was Joel's steroid appetite! Aside from costing pennies on the dollar as compared to microwave popcorn, there are no laboratory-invented ingredients here. Just coconut oil, whole-grain popcorn, and a little salt.

Instructions:

1. In a small sauce pan that has a lid, melt the coconut oil over medium-high heat.

2. Add in three popcorn kernels and cover with the lid.

3. Once the three kernels have popped, you know the oil is at the perfect temperature! Add in the remaining kernels quickly and replace the lid.

4. Once popping has slowed down significantly (you'll notice, I promise), remove the still-covered pan from heat.

5. Remove lid and salt to taste.

6. Serve immediately, or save in an airtight container at room temperature for 1-2 days.

Makes approximately 3 Cups

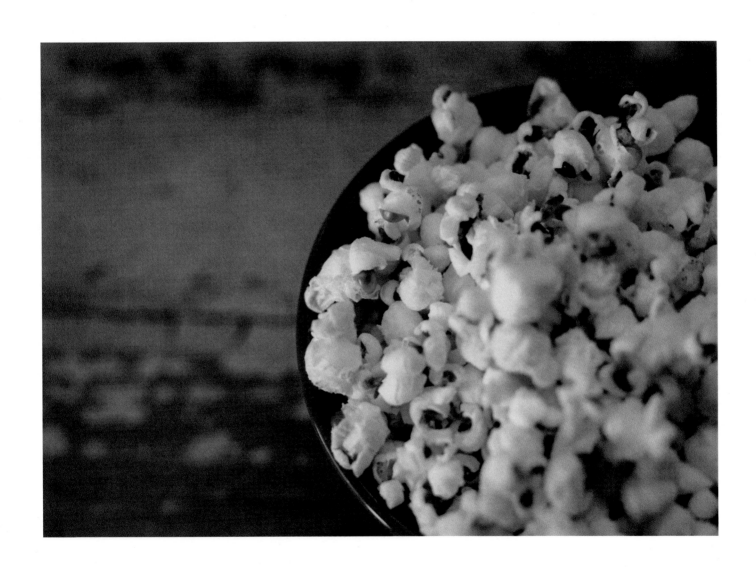

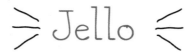 Jello

Ingredients:

2 Tablespoons beef gelatin powder

¼ Cup room temperature water

2 Cups organic, 1-ingredient juice (or fresh-squeezed, if you're feeling fancy)

If you're like me, you grew up with bright, jiggly jello from a box. So the thought of jello being good for you might make you stop and say "whaaaaaa?" And if we were talking about the neon powder from the 80's kids' childhood, I would indeed be off my rocker. Added sugar, food coloring, and artificial favors have zero benefits to a growing body—let alone a growing body fighting cancer! But you know what is super-beneficial? Beef gelatin. Thought to be good for bones, joints, digestion, hair, and fingernails, it is also soothing to the tummy—which is huge for chemo patients. Add to that the vitamins from real fruit juice and you've got yourself a winner.

Making jello cups from grass-fed beef gelatin takes the same amount of time as un-loading the dishwasher. I give such a weirdly specific example because that's how I timed it when I made jello for my sick kid just this week. I love knowing that when the only thing gentle enough is jello, it can still be helpful to my son's little body!

Note: I buy my gelatin in a 1-pound bag from NOW foods. There are a lot of great brands available, this is just the cheapest for me! Gelatin powder is available through most online health food websites, such as Thrive Market, iHerb, and Amazon, but is also at most local health food stores. For me, a bag will last almost a year. Also, this recipe multiplies really well. You can easily double or triple when the jello need is high!

Instructions:

1. In a small saucepan, heat the juice over medium-high heat.
2. While the juice is heating, add the water to a medium mixing bowl and sprinkle the gelatin over top.
3. As soon as the juice reaches a low boil, remove it from heat and pour it into the bowl with the gelatin.
4. Stir well to melt the gelatin into the juice.
5. Pour jello into small jars or a medium bowl, depending on if you like individual cups or scooped jello.
6. Refrigerate until set. This usually takes 4-5 hours.

Store in the refrigerator for up to 7-10 days.

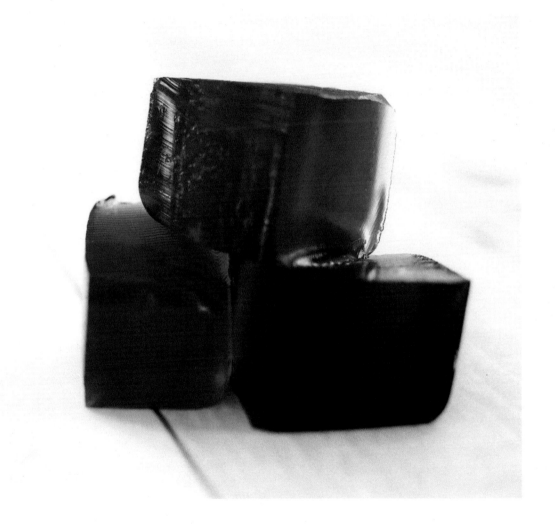

Veggies: Assemble! Pasta Sauce

Ingredients:

Two 14 oz. cans organic tomato sauce

½ Cup pureed butternut squash

¼ Cup pureed cauliflower

½ Cup packed fresh spinach

2 Tablespoons olive oil

1 teaspoon garlic powder

1 teaspoon dried oregano

½ teaspoon onion powder

½ teaspoon dried basil

1 teaspoon salt

1 Tablespoon maple syrup

Red pasta sauce is a staple on kids' menus in restaurants for a reason: they love it. This makes red sauce a great carrier for a myriad of other nutrient-packed veggies! Butternut squash, cauliflower, and even spinach fly under the radar when they hitchhike along with a plate of pasta with red sauce.

This recipe is easily doubled-- or even TRIPLED-- and freezes like a dream!

Instructions:

1. In a medium-sized saucepan or Dutch oven, add tomato sauce and spinach.
2. Bring to a simmer and cover the pan. Let cook on low heat for 10 minutes.
3. Remove from heat and use an immersion blender to puree until smooth.
4. Return to heat and add in all other ingredients.
5. Let simmer on low heat with the lid cock-eyed on the pan to allow steam out.
6. Simmer for 5 minutes.
7. Serve immediately or freeze in jars, allowing 1" headspace.

Makes about 2 ½ cups

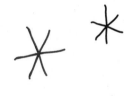

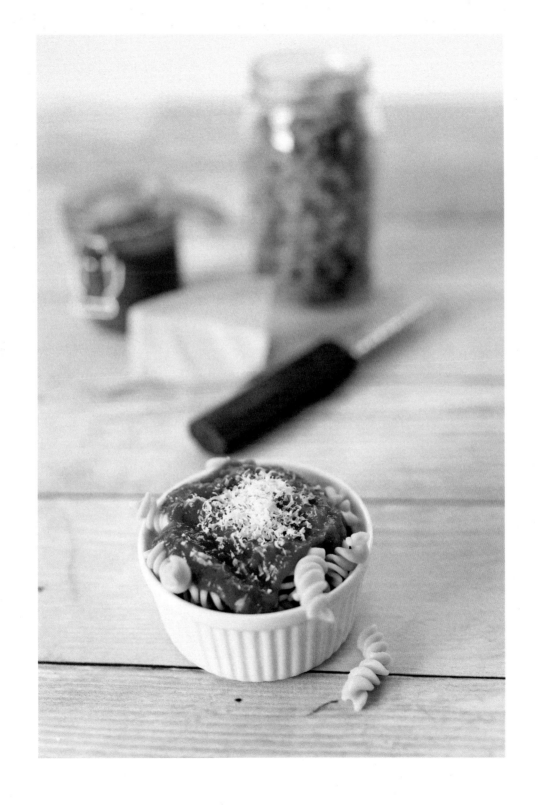

Pizza Grilled Cheese

Ingredients:

8 slices whole grain bread

4 slices mozzarella cheese

Butter

Veggies: Assemble! Sauce for dipping

So simple, so much fun! I truly feel like a rock star when I serve this up for my boys... Mostly because I tend to make it when I feel like I have nothing to feed hungry kids and its lunchtime RIGHT NOW. And then suddenly, I remember I can turn 4 ingredients I've got hanging around into a well-balanced lunch that makes the boys feel spoiled. Phew! Whole grains in the bread, calcium and protein in the cheese, and veggies for days in the dipping sauce. Last minute lunch? Nailed it!

Instructions:

1. Butter one side of each of the 8 slices of bread.

2. Place a slice of cheese between two slices, buttered side out.

3. Place each sandwich on a non-stick griddle or frying pan over medium-high heat.

4. Once the bottom is brown and the cheese looks a little melted, flip over the sandwiches.

5. Cook until the bottom is browned.

6. Remove the sandwiches from heat and cut in half to speed up the cooling.

7. Serve immediately with Veggies: Assemble! Sauce for dipping!

Serves 4

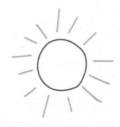

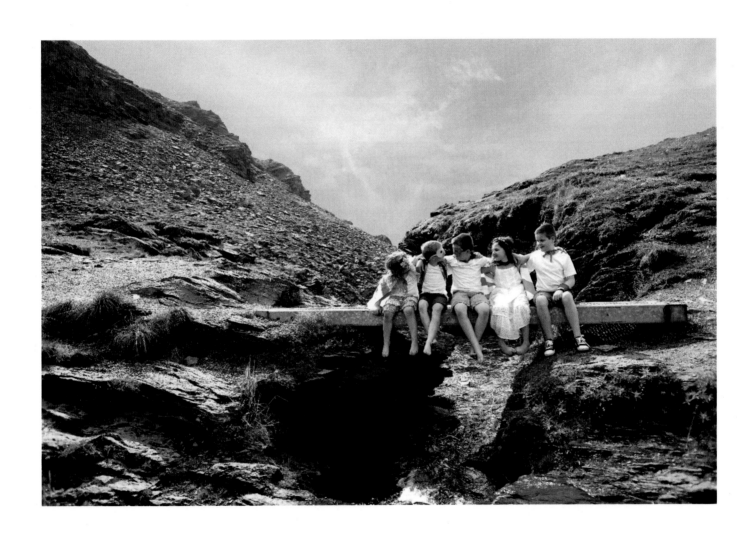

Cheesy Veggie Mini Meatloaves

Ingredients:

1 lb. ground meat (beef, wild game, or turkey)

1 Cup shredded cheese (we use cheddar, but most cheeses will work just fine!)

⅓ Cup breadcrumbs (made from the heel slice of our favorite bread on)

1 egg

½ to 1 Cup grated vegetables (carrot, onion, cauliflower, zucchini, squash, parsnip, potato, whatever you have around!)

Chemo causes tastes and appetites to ebb and flow. There will be times when your kiddo wants to eat nothing, and they lose a bit of weight. There are other times, like with steroids, when your kid wants to eat all the things and will put on some weight. There are times when ground meat will be completely out of the question, because of mouth sores or a sensitive digestive system. I did not give these to Joel much during treatment. But, those brothers? The ones dragged along to the hospital on a daily basis? The ones who were always hungry? They devoured these. And now I love feeding them to Joel as well while he begins his journey of survivorship. With his little body recovering from years of chemo, these mini-meatloaves provide protein and vitamins to be a superhero-worthy lunch!

Making the meatloaves mini cuts down on cook time in a big way. Plus, small food is just more fun for kids! My boys like these dipped in ranch.

Instructions:

1. Preheat the oven to 425 degrees.

2. Grease a 12 cup muffin tin.

3. Combine all ingredients in a medium-sized mixing bowl.

4. Mix well with your (washed) hands.

5. As evenly as you can, distribute the meat among the 12 muffin cups.

6. Bake for 15-17 minutes.

7. Let cool for 5 minutes and remove from the tin.

8. Serve immediately or freeze in Ziploc bags for up to 2 months.

Make 12 meatloaves.

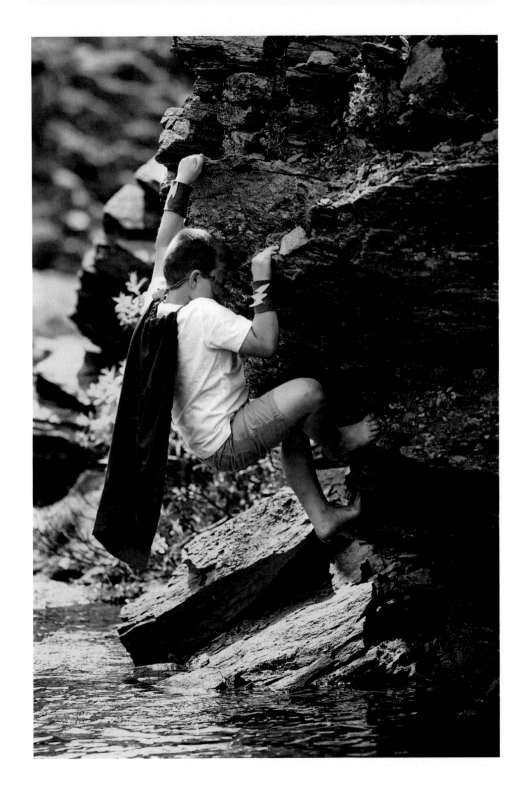

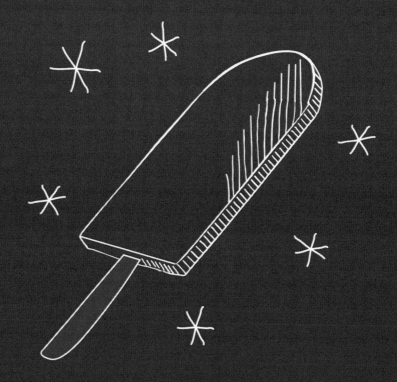

Sweet

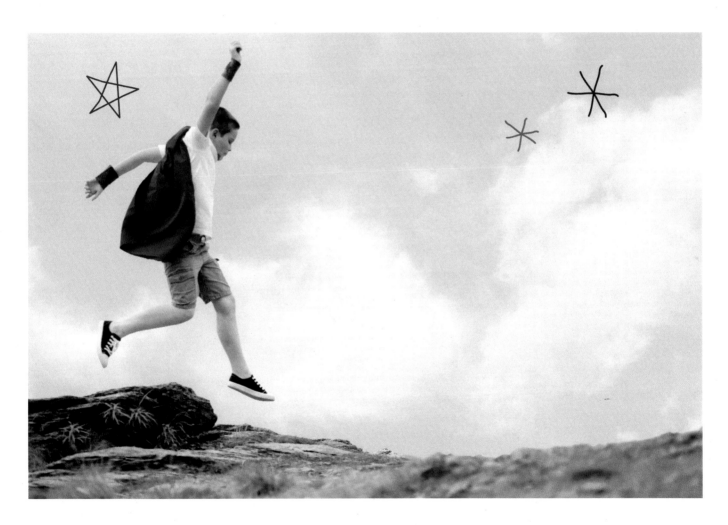

PB&J Popsicles

Ingredients:

¾ Cup Plain Whole Milk Yogurt

⅓ Cup peanut butter

⅓ cup pureed butternut squash

I Tablespoon honey

2 Cups of berries (strawberries are our favorite)

I teaspoon honey

Some things are just meant to be together: Heroes and capes; villains and plans of world domination; and peanut butter and jelly. Sore mouths are no match for this nutritious popsicle.

Instructions:

I. In a bowl, whisk yogurt, peanut butter, butternut squash and honey until smooth.

2. Evenly distribute among popsicle molds or smoothie pop containers.

3. In a blender, blend the strawberries and second tablespoon of honey until smooth. (If ANC is below 500, the berry sauce from works really well here!)

4. Evenly distribute the berry mixture over the peanut butter mixture.

5. Insert a knife in the popsicle molds to push the berries up into the peanut butter a little bit.

6. Freeze until needed, at least 4 hours.

7. Store in the freezer for up to 6 months.

Makes approximately 6-8 large popsicles

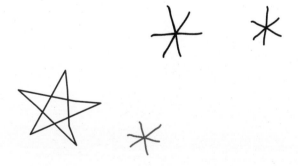

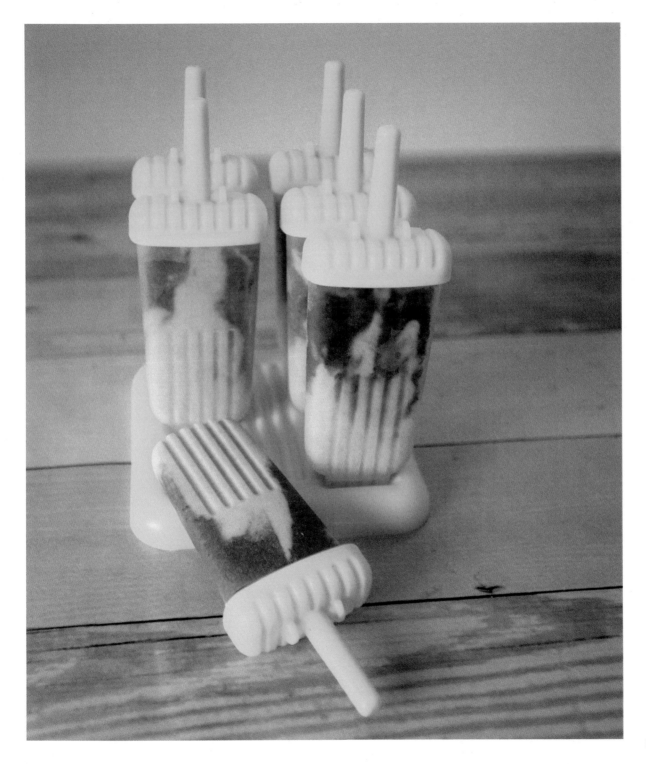

⇒ Cinnamon Roll Milk ⇐

Ingredients:

2 Cups whole milk

2 Tablespoons maple syrup

¼ teaspoon cinnamon

¼ teaspoon vanilla extract

If steroids are a part of your child's cancer treatment, then you are likely already on the offense to protect those growing bones. While great against leukemia, steroids can cause brittle bones and even osteoporosis later in life. This cinnamon roll milk is a delicious, comforting way to load your superhero with the vitamin D and calcium necessary to protect and build healthy bones—a must for leaping tall buildings in a single bound!

Instructions:

1. Combine all ingredients in a small sauce pan.

2. Heat over medium heat until steaming.

3. Serve immediately, or pour into an insulated thermos to be enjoyed later in the day.

☞ ** A dollop of whipped cream and a sprinkle of cinnamon makes this feel like an extra special treat!

Makes 2 cups

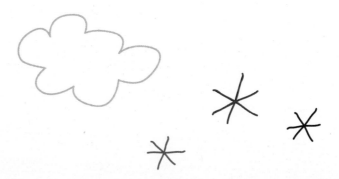

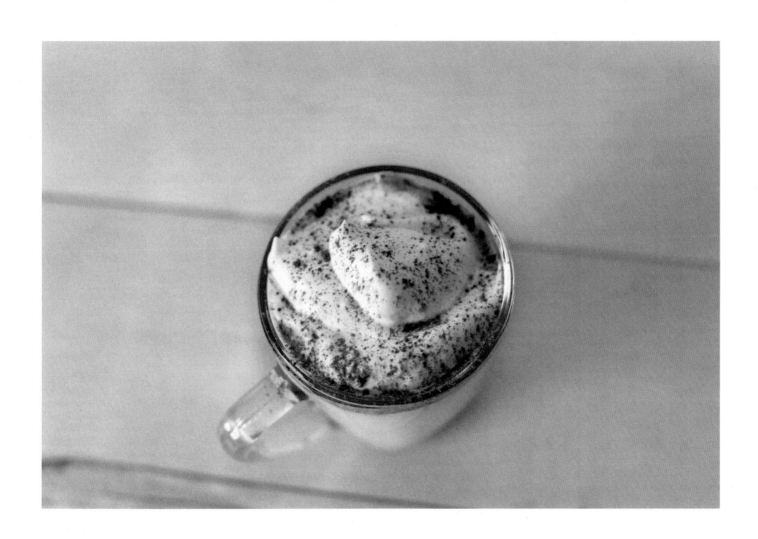

Cashew Butter Chocolate Chip Cookies

Ingredients:

1 ¼ Cup whole wheat flour

½ teaspoon baking soda

½ teaspoon salt

¾ Cup cashew butter

¾ Cup maple syrup

½ Cup butter (slightly colder than room temperature)

1 egg

1 teaspoon vanilla

½ Cup mini chocolate chips

These cookies were a little for the kids, but a whole lot for me. You see, I need to be able to make a plate of warm cookies for my kids, just so I can make every problem disappear—even if it's only for a moment. Chocolate chip cookies give me a feeling of empowerment: Yes, cancer stinks... but I can still make my kids' day with fresh cookies!

And fear not parents, these cookies don't bring a smile at the expense of nutrition. They are loaded with Iron-rich cashew butter, whole grains, and sweetened only with pure maple syrup.

Instructions:

1. Preheat the oven to 350 degrees F.
2. Using a stand mixer with a whisk attachment, or a handheld beater, mix together the butter, cashew butter, egg, maple syrup, and vanilla. Beat until smooth.
3. Add in the salt and baking soda and mix until well incorporated.
4. Using a big spoon, gently stir in the flour until *almost* completely combined.
5. Add in the chocolate chips and gently stir until evenly dispersed.
6. Drop spoonfuls of batter onto an ungreased cookie sheet.
7. Bake 12-15 minutes, or until lightly browned.
8. Let cool on the cookie sheet for a few minutes before transferring to a rack to cool completely.

Makes 15-20 cookies

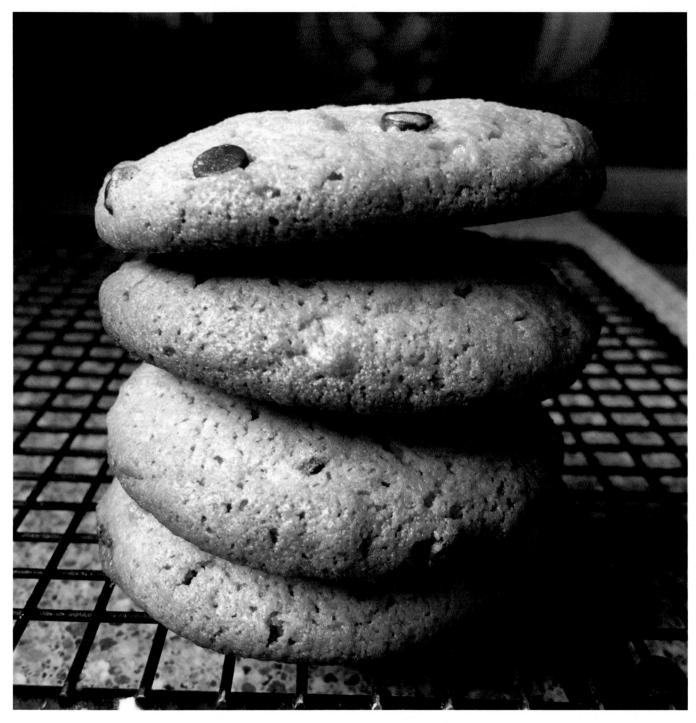

Yogurt Sundaes

Ingredients:

2 Cups plain, whole milk Greek yogurt

2 Tablespoons maple syrup

Chocolate Sauce

Berry Sauce

Mini Chocolate Chips

Sliced banana

Of my three boys, two love yogurt, one is hit-or-miss. Setting up a "build your own yogurt sundae" bar is our favorite way to guarantee yogurt is a hit. My favorite part is seeing the boys' eyes as big as saucers when they come downstairs for breakfast and see this spread laid out across the counter! Even my reluctant yogurt-eater can't help but enjoy his own creation.

Instructions:

1. In a small mixing bowl, stir together the yogurt and maple syrup.

2. Scoop yogurt into four small bowls.

3. Let the kids choose their own toppings and build amazing sundae creations!

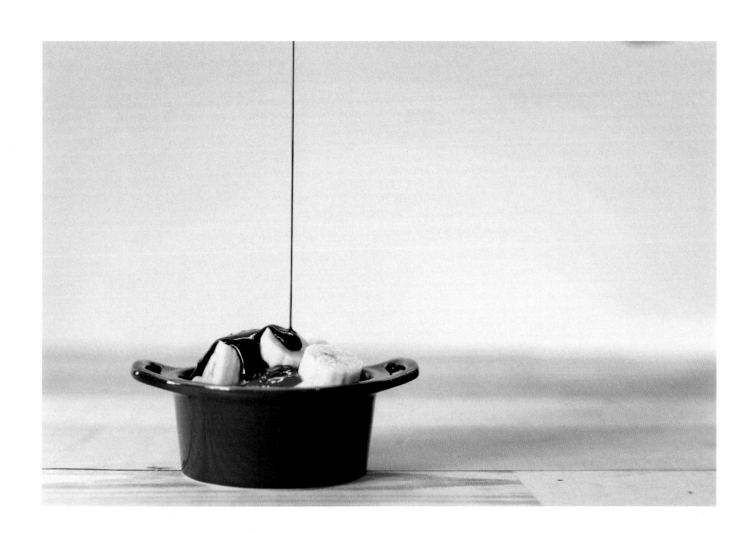

Chocolate Pudding

Ingredients:

4 large, ripe avocados, pitted and peeled

½ Cup unsweetened cocoa powder

¾ - 1 Cup pure maple syrup

1 Cup fresh spinach (omit if ANC is below 500)

Mmm, pudding… This was a fun way for Joel to load on the calories when weight gain was a must. Even now, I add this to school lunches because the dose of healthy fats keeps the boys' bellies full and happy until the very end of the day.

This same recipe can also be frozen into smoothie pop molds to make some amazingly chocolaty fudge-pops!

Instructions:

1. Place all ingredients into a food processor and blend until smooth. Alternatively, you can use an immersion blender.

2. Store in glass jars in the refrigerator for 7-10 days.

Makes about 5 cups.

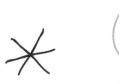

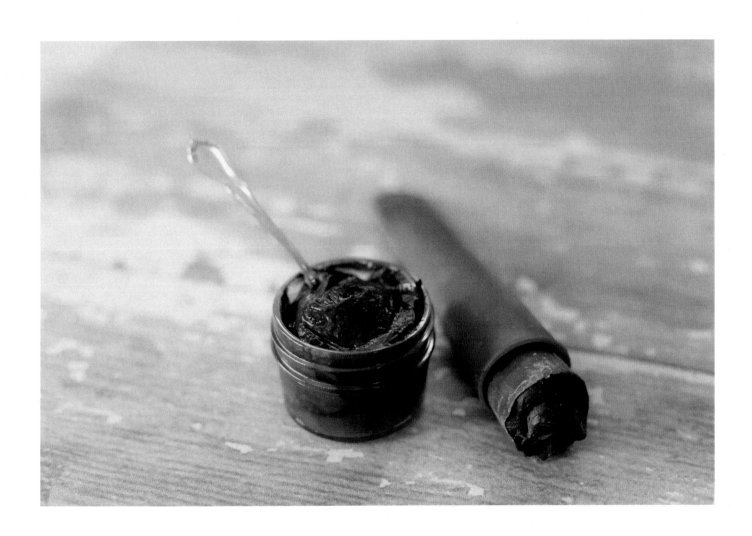

Orange Creamsicles

Ingredients:

3 oranges, peeled with a knife to remove most of the pith

½ Cup plain, whole milk yogurt

¼ Cup pureed cauliflower

1 Tablespoon honey

1 good splash of vanilla extract

Spellcheck is telling me "creamsicle" is not a word. But you and I both know it is. "Creamsicle" is just another way of saying "a summer afternoon so hot you try and slurp down your popsicle before it all drips onto the sidewalk." Am I right? And unlike the creamsicles from my childhood, this one not only tastes like sunshine, but it also nourishes hard-working superheroes.

Instructions:

1. Combine all ingredients in a blender and blend until smooth.

2. Pour into smoothie pop molds or popsicle molds, leaving half an inch at the top.

3. Freeze 5 hours or overnight.

Makes about 6 popsicles

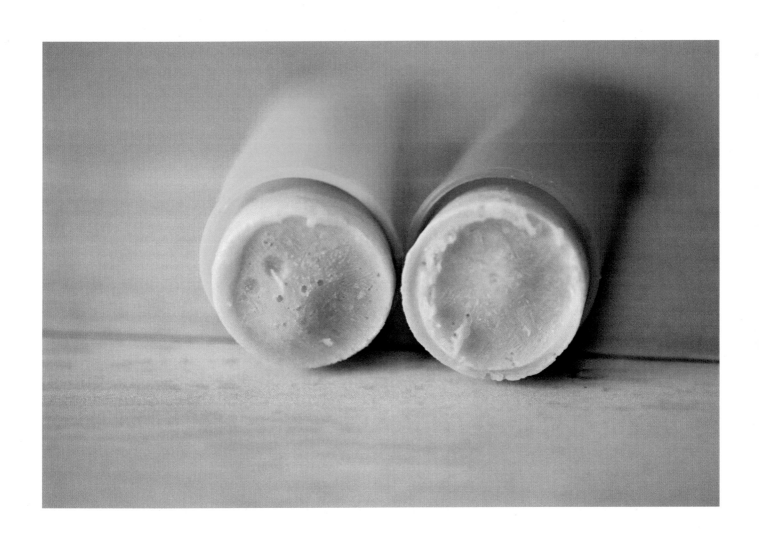

Creamy Hot Chocolate

Ingredients:

1 ½ Cups whole milk

⅓ Cup pureed sweet potato

Chocolate syrup to taste (I use almost ¼ cup, but my husband prefers it much lighter. To each their own. But he's wrong.)

A snow day in a mug, with more nutritional benefits than you'd have time to read. Well, you'd probably have time, but you would get bored with such a long list and just want to get on to drinking this creamy, delicious, mug of goodness.

Instructions:

1. Combine all ingredients in a small saucepan.

2. Stir with a whisk while heating on medium-low.

3. Serve immediately (with freshly whipped cream!) or put into a thermos for transport to the hospital.

Serves 2

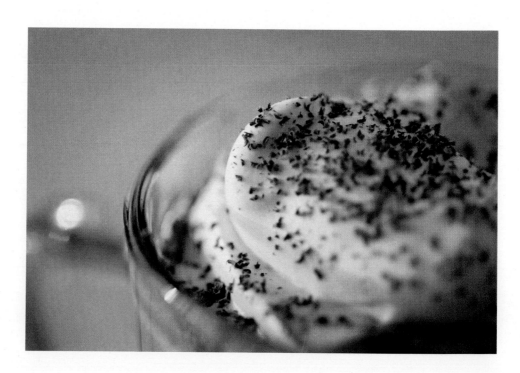

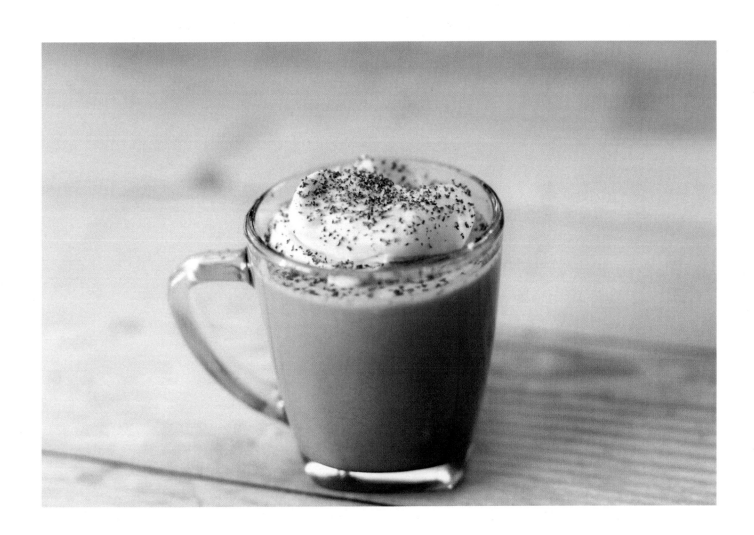

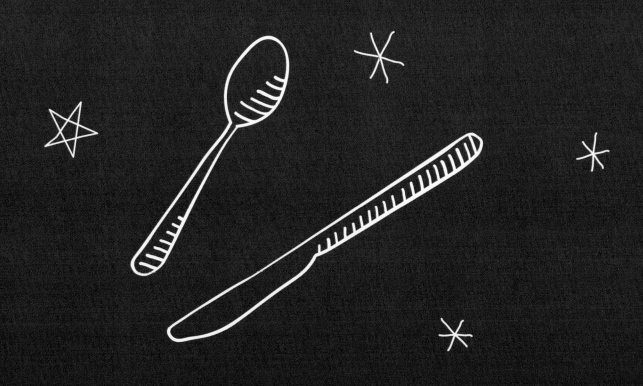

Dips and Spreads

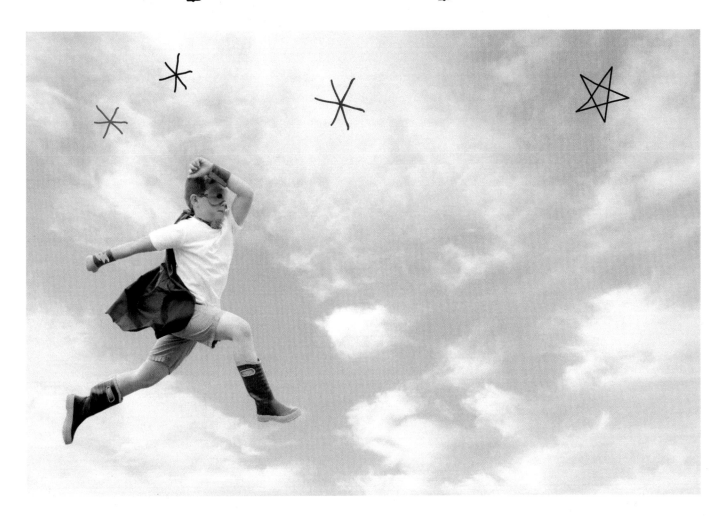

Chocolate Almond Butter

Ingredients:

½ Cup Almond Butter

⅓ Cup High-Quality Chocolate Chips

This chocolate spread seamlessly replaced the store-bought version in our home... partly because it's so stinkin' delicious, and partly because the boys love how we make it ourselves!

Instructions:

1. Fill a small saucepan half-full with water and bring to a boil. Place a small mixing bowl over the pan as a lid. (This is your make-shift double boiler!)

2. Place all ingredients in the bowl and stir until melted and combined.

3. Store in a glass container in the pantry for a week, or the refrigerator for a month.

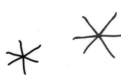 **Have fun and get creative with this by swapping out different nut butters (or even sunflower butter) and chocolates! Some fun combinations include walnut and dark chocolate, cashew and semi-sweet chocolate, or peanut butter and milk chocolate.

Makes ¾ Cup

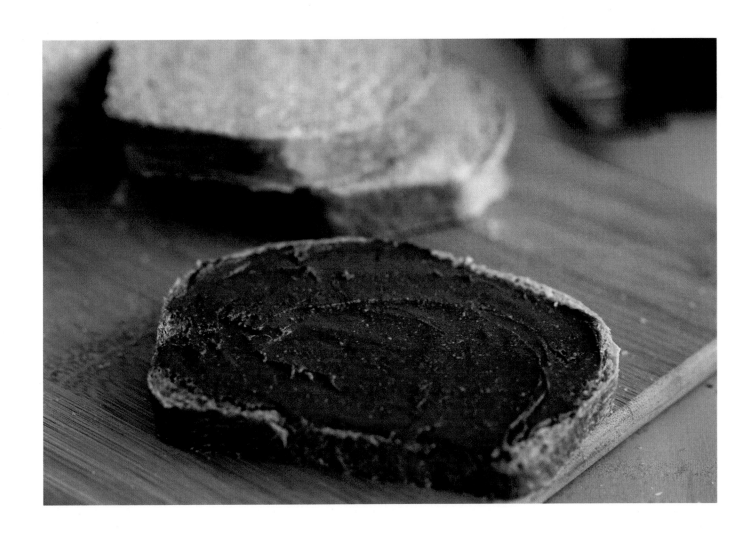

Ranch Dip

Ingredients:

For the Ranch seasoning-

I Tablespoon dried dill weed

2 teaspoons garlic powder

2 teaspoons onion powder

I teaspoon salt

I teaspoon pepper

For the dip-

I Cup sour cream

½ Cup mayonnaise (I like homemade mayo the best, but during chemo, shelf-stable is the safe choice. Try and find an organic brand with minimal ingredients, like Chosen Foods or Sir Kensington brand.)

I Tablespoon ranch seasoning

With no whack-a-do ingredients, you'll feel pretty great about letting your kid have a little carrot with their ranch! A child's desire to dunk their veggies in dip is actually their brilliant little body craving the fats necessary to absorb the vitamins in the vegetables. And, let's be real, ranch dip cuts whining over veggies down by about 90%.

Instructions:

(For the seasoning)

1. Combine all ingredients in a small jar.

2. Store at room temperature in a small jar for up to I year.

(For the Dip)

1. Combine the dip ingredients in a small bowl.

2. Stir.

3. Store in the refrigerator in an air-tight glass container for up to two weeks.

Makes I ½ Cups of dip.

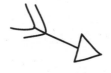
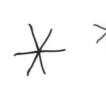

Cream Cheese Dip

Ingredients:

½ Cup cream cheese at room temperature

¼ Cup Greek yogurt

2 Tablespoons pure maple syrup

¼ teaspoon vanilla

Instructions:

1. Combine all ingredients in a small mixing bowl.

2. Whisk until smooth.

3. Serve with bananas, strawberries, beet pancakes, or banana muffins!

4. Store in an airtight container in the refrigerator for up to two weeks.

Makes approximately 1 Cup

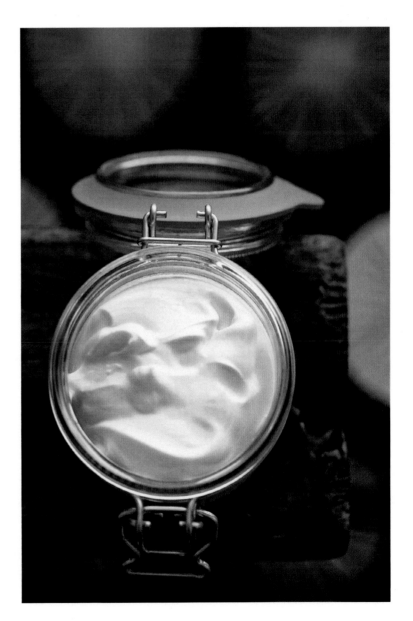

10-Minute Cheese Sauce

Ingredients:

2 Tablespoons whole wheat flour

2 Tablespoons butter

I Cup whole milk

I ½ Cups freshly shredded cheddar cheese

¼ - ½ teaspoon salt

I grew up in the dairy state, so perhaps I am a little biased about the super powers of cheese... But let's just be honest with ourselves: what would you NOT eat that has cheese sauce poured all over it? Yeah. Exactly. And since this cheese sauce is actually made from cheese, you don't have to cringe about this being the reason your superhero eats roasted broccoli! Unlike with the plastic-ish, bright orange, never-goes-bad, usually served at a shady skating rink stuff we also call "cheese sauce." Yikes.

We love this sauce with roasted veggies, of course, but it is also amazing with mini meatloaves, Baked potatoes, and Squashed and Scrambled Eggs.

Instructions:

1. Melt the butter in a saucepan over medium heat. Whisk in the flour and cook for I minute.

2. Slowly pour in the milk and continue to whisk while it thickens. This takes about 3-4 minutes. Don't stop whisking here, we don't want any lumps!

3. Turn off the heat and add in the freshly shredded cheese (pre-shredded has a coating that can keep it from melting well). Stir in the cheese with a spoon until smooth.

4. Add in salt to taste and stir.

5. Serve immediately.

Makes about 2 Cups sauce.

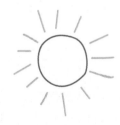

Cinnamon Peanut Butter Dip

Ingredients:

½ Cup Greek yogurt

3 Tablespoons peanut butter

2 teaspoons pure maple syrup

¼ teaspoon cinnamon

This dip is great with apples and bananas! We've also used it spread on bread for a filling snack.

Instructions:

1. Combine all ingredients in a small mixing bowl.

2. Whisk until smooth.

3. Serve with apples, pears, bananas, or crackers!

4. Store in an airtight container in the fridge for up to 2 weeks.

Makes approximately ¾ Cup.

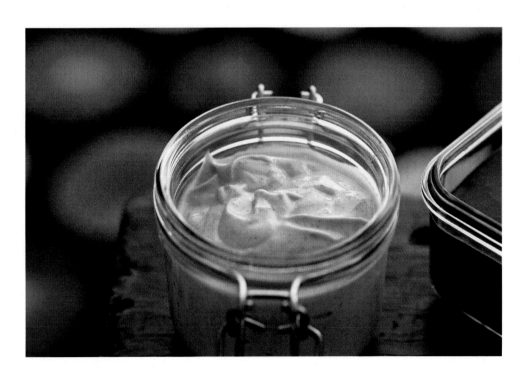

Chocolate Sauce

Ingredients:

1 Cup pure maple syrup

⅓ Cup Unsweetened cocoa

A Splash of vanilla extract

A sore mouth is no match for a tall, cold glass of chocolate milk! This chocolate sauce has three simple ingredients and takes just a few minutes to throw together, making chocolate milk and hot chocolates into a simple and wholesome treat. Childhood: 1 Cancer: 0.

Instructions:

1. Using either a jar and microwave or a saucepan and stovetop, heat the maple syrup to a little bit warmer than room temperature.

2. Add the cocoa powder and stir until completely combined.

3. Add in the vanilla and stir again.

4. Store in a jar in the refrigerator for up to a month.

Makes about 1 ¼ Cup of sauce.

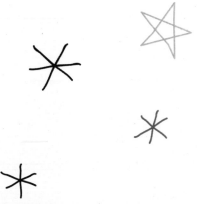

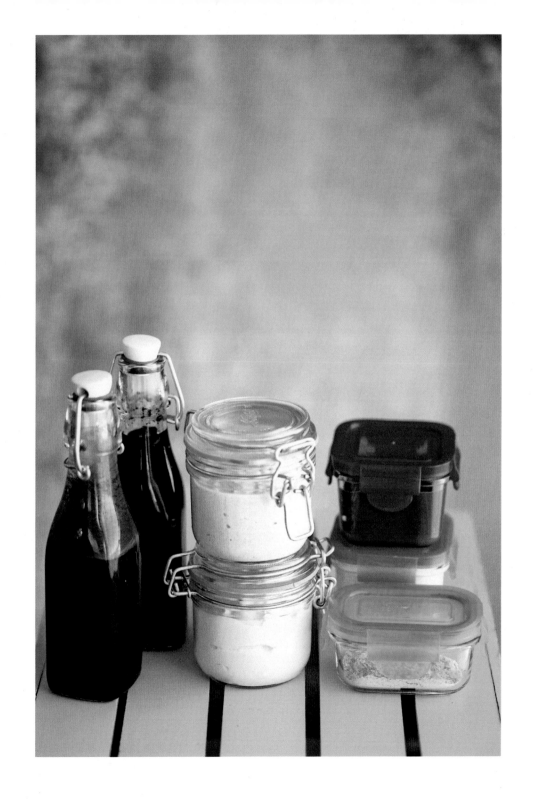

Berry Sauce

Ingredients:

5 Cup Blueberries,
(raspberries, cherries,
blackberries, strawberries)
fresh or frozen

¾ Cup Pure Maple syrup

¾ Cup water

2 Cups Fresh Spinach

A great way to use up berries that are almost to the end of their usefulness, this sauce brings fruit back into the picture when fresh fruit is a no-go. And (kids, look away) this is packed with a hefty dose of greens!

Instructions:

1. Combine all ingredients except for spinach in a saucepan over medium-high heat.

2. Bring to a simmer and reduce heat to medium-low.

3. Using a potato masher or fork, smash the berries every few minutes while they simmer.

4. Continue simmering and smashing for about 10 minutes, or until the sauce has the consistency of runny jam.

5. Add in the spinach and cook for 5 more minutes.

6. Using an immersion blender, blend the sauce until smooth.

7. Store in glass jars in the refrigerator for 3 weeks, or freeze (allowing 1-inch headspace in the jar) for up to a year.

Makes Approximately 5 Cups

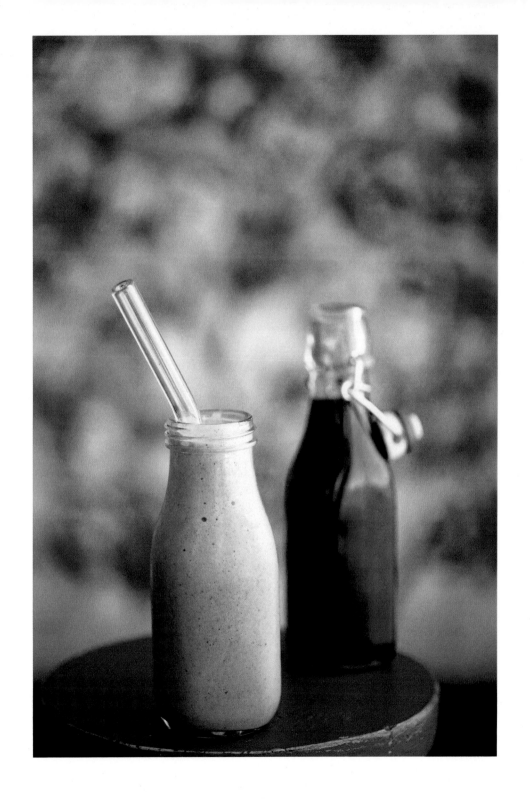

To **Willy**, the love of my life, my best friend, my biggest encouragement, and the one who taught me to be adventurous with food.

To **Nathan**, **Joel**, and **Eric**, my inspirations, cheerleaders, survivors, taste-testers, and joys.

To **Leslie**, my teammate in this project. Your photography is what made this book.

To **Tonya**, my proofreader and source of encouragement

To **all the many friends and family** who kept me trucking and pushing to get this book made.

To **all my recipe testers**, who tested and shaped and brought out the best in my recipes.

To the **doctors, nurses, and hospital staff** who brought the beauty and care that made cancer bearable.

To **all of our church family** at Wasilla Bible Church who never let us be abandoned in our time of sickness.

To **Fronteras Spanish Immersion School** who loved on us and always saved a seat for Joel.

To the **Cancer Community**. You are all my heroes.

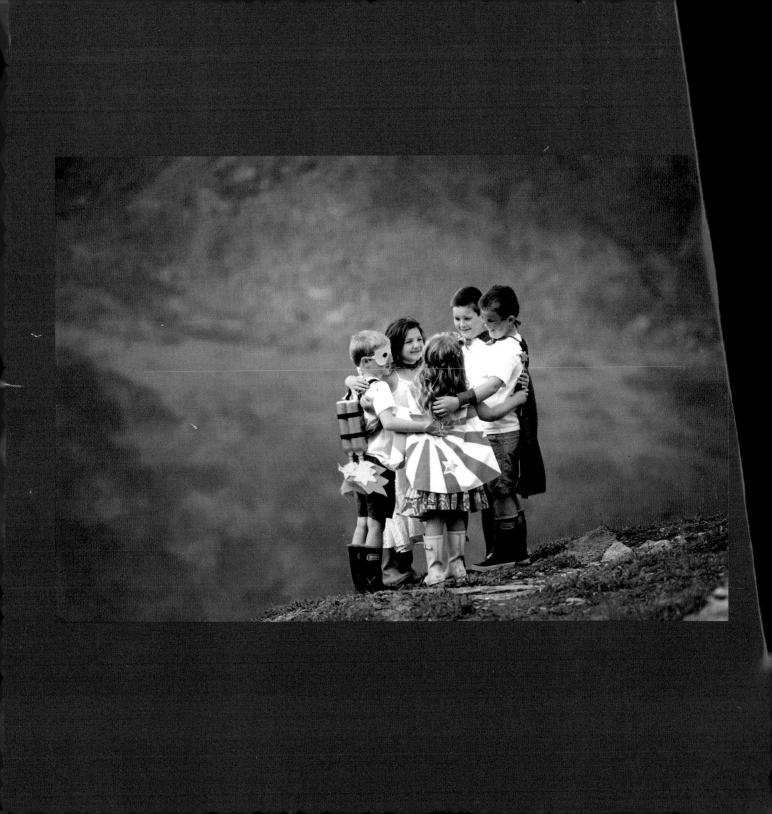